Addiction Free Pain Management

Recovery Guide

Managing Pain and Medication in Recovery

Developed by Stephen F. Grinstead
Foreword by Terence T. Gorski

Based on the Gorski-CENAPS® Model

Additional copies are available from the publisher:
Herald House/Independence Press
P.O. Box 390
Independence, MO 64051-0390
Phone: 1-800-767-8181 or (816) 521-3015

For training contact:
The CENAPS® Corporation
17900 Dixie Highway
Homewood, IL 60430
Phone: (708) 799-5000

Table of Contents

Foreword by Terence T. Gorski

Anyone with a chronic pain disorder needs information about how to manage their pain without becoming addicted to pain medication. People who are recovering from addiction need to know how to manage their pain conditions without relapsing. This recovery guide provides this information in a clear, concise, and easy-to-understand way.

Recovering people are at risk of relapsing as a result of an illness or injury resulting in severe pain. These relapses are often caused because recovering people don't have accurate information about pain, pain disorders, pain management, and the appropriate role of pain medication.

I've been concerned about pain management in recovery since 1970. One of my clients—I'll call him Roy—went into the hospital for routine surgery to remove his infected appendix. I did the normal addiction counseling with him. I helped him to understand that he could become addicted to pain medications. I advised him to talk openly with his doctor. I set up a plan for people from his Twelve-Step support group to be actively involved during his recuperation from the surgery. I thought this would be enough—but I was wrong.

Roy began having problems even before his surgery. His fear of using pain medications made him anxious about relapse. When he tried to talk with his doctor about his concerns, the doctor put him off and assured him that the anesthetics and pain medications were "non-addictive." Roy knew this wasn't true, but his doctor wouldn't even discuss it with him. Roy asked me to talk with his doctor, but the doctor would never return my phone calls.

People in his Twelve-Step group weren't very helpful. Some of them told him that if he used any pain medications at all it would mean he was in relapse. Others just told him not to worry about it and "turn it over." He also got the message that if he had a solid recovery program he'd be fine. Well, Roy didn't feel fine; he was scared to death. He mistakenly believed this fear was the result of not having a "good enough recovery program."

Roy was admitted to the hospital the night before surgery. When he was given a sleeping pill, he tried to refuse. The nurses told him if he didn't take the sleeping pill, there could be problems in the surgery the next day. Not knowing what to do, Roy gave in and took the sleeping pill. A part of him felt guilty about using the sleeping pill. Another part of him was relieved. At least he'd be able to get some sleep if he took the pill. He wasn't sure that he'd get any sleep if he didn't have the pill to help him sleep. When he awoke in the morning, he felt groggy and irritable. But he was immediately given sedatives, which calmed him down and spaced him out. He really liked how those preoperative medications made him feel. Roy was kept heavily sedated until three o'clock in the afternoon when he was finally taken into surgery.

After the operation he began to experience progressive pain, but he didn't ask for pain medication. He believed he could "tough it out." He was fearful that if he used any pain medication at all, it would mean that he had relapsed into his addiction. When the pain became unbearable, he gave in and asked for pain medication. He felt guilty but he just couldn't stand the pain. The medication they gave him at first was not enough to take care of the pain so they increased the type and amount. He was kept heavily medicated on narcotic injections for two days. Each injection put him in a narcotic stupor for about twenty minutes, and as he came back to normal consciousness the pain started up again. By the time he could get another shot in four hours the pain was once again unbearable. Then he was suddenly cut off and discharged with a prescription for thirty "pain pills," which he was supposed to take four times a day for four or five days.

The night after Roy got home, he started feeling the symptoms of narcotic withdrawal and started craving the drugs. He took the pain pills more frequently than prescribed. The pain was real and he needed relief. Then the alcohol cravings started. He began to panic because the pain was still severe, he was craving alcohol, and his pills were running out. He believed the pain pills were his only way to get through the pain without drinking.

He went to his family doctor and got some additional pain medication. During the postoperative visit with the surgeon he also got another prescription. About ten days after his surgery he was home alone. He took four pain pills to help him sleep. Then he started thinking about drinking. When the alcohol craving set in, he drove to the liquor store and bought a fifth of bourbon. He came home and started drinking. The next week he was back in the hospital for "surgical complications." In the hospital he went into alcohol and drug withdrawal. The doctor referred him back to the addiction treatment program. The first time I knew anything was wrong was when I got a call to go see Roy in a medical bed.

At that time I knew there must be a better way to help people prepare for the trauma of surgery and to get through postoperative pain without relapse. Pain management was a newly emerging concept. There just wasn't much information about how to help recovering people deal with postoperative pain.

As the population of baby boomers started to age, many of them got into recovery from alcoholism and other drug addictions. As they have aged, they began to experience many illnesses that are accompanied by severe and chronic pain. Some of these painful medical conditions, such as AIDS, liver disease, and hepatitis, can be directly caused by addictive alcohol or drug use. Other illnesses are the result of poor health care and the heavy abuse of the body that often accompanies chronic addiction. Some of these illnesses are related to the normal problems associated with aging.

Over the years I've known many people who suffered from AIDS. Some of them relapsed as a result of the serious illnesses and pain caused by conditions related to AIDS. Others relapsed because they couldn't deal with the pain, uncertainty, and fear. A few even committed suicide. I've also had several friends who were suffering from terminal cancer, relapsed, and committed suicide as a result of mismanaging the pain. As I am writing this introduction, another friend of mine is in a rehabilitation program dealing with a relapse that was triggered by serious chronic heart disease complicated by progressive back pain caused by an old injury.

Although the theme of pain as a relapse trigger came up over and over again in relapse prevention training and clinical consultation, there was no comprehensive approach that integrated effective pain management techniques with effective addiction treatment methods. I am excited to say that this is no longer the case.

Steve Grinstead has spent many years studying pain and its impact on recovery and relapse. His model integrates the principles of Twelve-Step recovery, biopsychosocial addiction treatment, and relapse prevention. It's been a pleasure working with Steve. I've learned a great deal from him as we worked together to organize his knowledge and expertise with pain management. The result was the development of the Addiction-Free Pain Management (APM) System. APM is a practical and nononsense model for helping people manage pain without becoming addicted and without relapsing if they are in recovery.

All recovering people should learn the basics of Addiction-Free Pain Management (APM) so they will be prepared if they experience an illness or injury that causes pain. All addiction treatment programs should have specialty programs for helping recovering people prepare for surgery, deal with acute pain problems resulting from surgery and injuries, and to deal with chronic pain that is related to many illnesses and serious injuries.

Steve's work gives me hope. There is now something we can do to help recovering people deal with pain in a realistic and practical way without relapsing. This method can also be applied in pain clinics to help people manage pain disorders without becoming addicted. This recovery guide will give you the best information available about how to manage pain without becoming addicted or relapsing. You'll find that this information is presented in a clear, interesting, and easy-to-understand way. Most importantly, if you choose to use the methods described in this book, you'll find that they work. You'll discover it is possible to find relief from severe chronic pain while staying in recovery from addiction.

Terence T. Gorski

Acknowledgments

As anyone who has done it before can tell you, writing a book takes the commitment and cooperation of many people. There are several people who have helped me who deserve special acknowledgment for making this book possible. I want to thank Terence T. Gorski, founder and president of the CENAPS® Corporation, who helped me to conceptualize and bring this book into its final form with his critical analysis, comments, and suggestions, as well as writing the foreword.

The following people also helped me immensely. Without their outstanding efforts I never would have learned to manage my own pain disorder and this book would not have been possible. Some of the professionals who gave so freely of their own expertise are: Dr. Kenneth Goranson, an orthopedic surgeon who was willing to support an alternative treatment approach; Dr. Diana Martin, a chiropractor who taught me many valuable pain reduction tools; and Ms. Lynn Wiese, a psychotherapist who helped me to look at the emotional and psychological components of my own pain.

I also want to thank Ellen Gruber-Grinstead for her assistance in editing and formatting this book and Barbara Block, LCSW, who provided me with encouragement and her own clinical expertise. I especially want to thank my private practice clients who helped to enrich this book through their own APM journey.

Stephen F. Grinstead

Chapter One

From Victimization to Empowerment

A Roadmap for Using this Book

Some of you may be reading this book because you have a chronic pain condition and are looking for help. Others may be family members who are living with someone in chronic pain and you want to learn how to help your loved ones. Some of you may be in recovery from chemical dependency and are afraid you might relapse over a pain condition. Maybe you're not in recovery, but you have chronic pain and want to avoid becoming chemically dependent. Or you may be in chronic pain and have begun to either abuse or become dependent on your pain medication, which may be causing a variety of problems in your life. Whatever the reason, I want you to know that it is possible to escape the bonds of pain and addiction. I want to help you recognize a potential problem and develop an effective solution.

I am writing this recovery guide directly to those of you with chronic pain. Whoever you are, I want you to know there is hope if you have chronic pain and fear ineffective pain management, chemical dependency, or relapse. I also hope that family members or others who do not have chronic pain will benefit from reading this book and be able to understand from the point of view of those who have chronic pain.

The best way to get the greatest benefit from this book is to thoroughly read and understand the first four chapters. As you read these chapters be aware of your thinking and your feelings. It's also helpful to keep a notebook or journal close by as you read so you can write about your reactions to what you are learning.

> You Can Find Freedom
> From the Bondage of Pain
> Without Becoming Addicted or
> Without Relapsing to Addiction

When you get to the end of chapter four you should have a copy of the *Addiction-Free Pain Management (APM) Workbook* to use as you read the remainder of this book. Starting with chapter five, I explain the APM process by describing each exercise in the APM workbook and how two of my patients, Donna and Matt, used the APM process and completed each of the exercises. They experienced what I hope you can obtain by doing this work—freedom from the bondage of pain!

Looking at the Problem

> Getting out of the problem
> and into the solution

Before finding the solution, you need to look at the problem of pain. Chronic pain is a serious health concern confronting many people today. Pain is often disabling and for many of you there are few safe alternatives when seeking help. As a result, you may end up suffering or developing an addiction to the medications you are using to help manage your pain. Many people in chemical dependency recovery can relapse and may even die from their addiction as a result of an untreated—or mistreated—chronic pain condition.

The Roadblock Called Denial

If you don't know you have a problem it can be extremely difficult to find a solution. Many people I have worked with have a mistaken belief that "I can't be addicted because I'm in pain and a doctor gave me the medication." This can be a type of denial. If you have been abusing or have become addicted to your medication you will experience life-damaging consequences. If you're in denial, you won't be able to see those problems.

> ## Four Levels of Denial
> - Lack of Information
> - Conscious Defensiveness
> - Unconscious Defense Mechanism
> - Delusional System

There are four levels of denial. The first is a **lack of information** about addiction. The previous example shows this first level—the mistaken belief that because a doctor prescribed the medication, there won't be an addiction problem. The solution here is to be open to education and information about addiction. It's important for you to learn as much as possible about chemical dependency, pain disorders, and effective pain management.

The second level of denial is **conscious defensiveness**. You know that something is wrong, but you don't want to look at the problem and face the pain of knowing. The solution is to recognize that there is an inner conflict occurring where one part of you knows there's a problem, but another part doesn't want to admit it. To resolve this conflict you must be willing to listen to the part that knows the truth and take action. The old saying, "The truth will set you free," is certainly relevant in this case.

The third level is denial as an **unconscious defense mechanism**. You get to this level when you have stayed in the inner conflict, mentioned above, and the defensive voice keeps winning. Once this happens, denial becomes an unconscious defense mechanism. The solution is much more difficult. It usually takes an outside intervention, or what is called a motivational crisis, to break through this defense and allow you to know the truth and start addressing the problem. For some of my patients this motivational crisis was generated when their treating physicians became concerned about their use/abuse of pain medication. For others it was family members intervening and urging them to seek help.

The fourth level is denial as a **delusional system**, which is the toughest level to address. Terence Gorski describes this delusion as "a mistaken belief that is firmly held to be true despite convincing evidence that it is not true." If your denial were at this level, you probably would not be reading this book. People at this level of denial usually need long-term psychotherapy to resolve their delusional system.

I will discuss more about denial management in chapter seven. For an excellent resource on denial, you can read the *Denial Management Counseling Professional Guide* and the *Denial Management Counseling Workbook,* written by Terence T. Gorski and Stephen F. Grinstead.

Hitting the Depression Wall

Many people with chronic pain frequently become depressed due to living with undertreated or mistreated pain symptoms. This process starts when your thinking and emotions begin to become problematic. When your thinking becomes irrational or dysfunctional and you start mismanaging your feelings, you often have urges to indulge in self-defeating, impulsive, or compulsive behaviors to cope with your depression. This in turn affects your relationships with others.

The Pitfalls of Isolation and Enabling

Some people may become isolated and believe they can handle life without any help, or they may become increasingly dependent on others to take care of them. Either style can worsen their depression. This caretaking by others may be enabling the depressed person to continue ineffective behaviors and maintaining his or her role as a victim. Some of you may need to have treatment for depression. An effective depression management treatment plan includes cognitive behavioral therapy and possibly an antidepressant medication. The role of antidepressant medications is discussed in chapter three where I describe the APM *medication management components.*

The important thing to remember is that you need to be able to recognize and admit you have a problem before you can work on an effective solution. Typically you will need help—

a support network for instance—to work through any denial or depression issues in order to develop an effective recovery and pain management program, but be careful who you choose to help you. Sometimes self-help support people and health-care providers can become part of the problem.

Misguided "Helpers"

> Don't take nothin'—no matter what!

This statement can be heard frequently if you attend Alcoholics Anonymous (AA) or Narcotic Anonymous (NA) meetings. The message is, if you don't use any alcohol or other drugs you are clean and sober and will experience the promises of recovery, but if you take *anything,* "you've blown it — you've relapsed."

In most cases those words are good counsel for people recovering from chemical dependency. However, when the *nothin'* includes medication prescribed by a knowledgeable physician for a legitimate condition, those words could actually lead you to a relapse. Some examples of medications that are often prescribed to people in recovery include antidepressants, anti-anxiety medication, or pain medication. As a caution to members, AA's central office produced a pamphlet emphasizing that sponsors and others were "not to play doctor," and that sometimes people in recovery need to take *appropriate* medication.

> Dave's Story

Several years ago I had a client named Dave who fell victim to the "Don't take nothin'" message. Dave was a 19-year-old construction worker who had injured himself at work and was taking pain medication. He also suffered from a condition called bipolar (manic/depressive) disorder and was using alcohol and speed to self-medicate that condition. Dave was arrested for possession and being under the influence of methamphetamine. He was sent to the drug diversion program where I was the clinical supervisor.

When my counseling staff told me about Dave's pain condition, I met with him and gave him a referral to an addiction medicine specialist. This doctor put Dave on Celebrex, a non-narcotic anti-inflammatory medication, for his pain and a combination of Lithium and Prozac for his bipolar disorder. Dave was happy to be getting effective pain management help as well as relief for his bipolar condition. He was also becoming excited about being clean and sober. He started going to AA meetings and soon got a sponsor. Unfortunately, Dave's sponsor told him he wasn't really clean and sober because he was mood-altering with his medication.

Dave really wanted to be clean and sober so he listened to his sponsor and quit all his medication. I received a call a few weeks later from Dave's pregnant young wife telling me that Dave had killed himself in a manic episode. This did not have to happen! But well-meaning self-help people are not the only problem.

You're just drug seeking.

Problems with health-care providers usually occur in one of two ways. The first example is when the treatment provider decides that because you are an "addict" they won't prescribe *any* narcotic medication and end up treating you as "drug seeking." When consulting with other treatment professionals I try to explain to them that the person in pain is not "drug seeking," he or she is really seeking pain relief.

The other example is the doctor who thanks you for your honesty and is willing to prescribe narcotic medication but does not fully understand addiction or recovery. The doctor might say something like "We'll be careful." This lack of understanding can very well be a setup if you do not have an effective medication management plan in place.

Linda's Story

Linda, another client of mine, was referred to my private practice by her doctor for relapse prevention and pain management treatment planning. Linda had a past history of Vicodin addiction, which eventually led to her arrest for forging prescriptions. She had been in recovery for five years and was doing quite well with alternative pain management help from her doctor. Unfortunately, Linda started experiencing a significant increase in her pain and was afraid of needing narcotic medication.

I helped Linda and her doctor develop a pain medication management plan that included interventions for Linda's frequent pain flair-ups. This plan was working well until Linda's doctor was on vacation and she experienced an intense pain flair-up. She followed her backup plan that we developed. Because it was late on a Saturday night she went to the local hospital emergency room. She explained her situation to the staff and asked if anyone on staff was familiar with recovery and addiction—no one admitted to any knowledge.

Linda was put in an examination room where she waited for more than an hour. Finally, she got up to see what was taking so long and overheard the staff nurse telling the doctor that "We have another one of those damn drug seekers in room three." Linda was hurt and angry that they were talking about her like that and tried to explain her situation to the doctor. She even showed the doctor her emergency plan that we had developed with her doctor. This emergency room doctor told her that her doctor was not on staff at this hospital and that he was not willing to prescribe the medication on the plan. He did give her a prescription for Vicodin, which she fortunately tore up when she got home.

This story had a much happier ending. Linda called me and I referred her to another physician who not only helped her immediate pain flair-up but also discovered that all she needed was a simple surgical procedure that would stop this from happening again. Today Linda is still clean and sober and virtually pain free.

> ## You must have a plan.

What is especially true if you are in recovery for prescription medication, alcohol, or other drug dependency is that you must be very careful when using any mood-altering (psychoactive) medication. The most common problems occur with pain medication. You need to use caution, have a plan, and have support.

Over the past two decades I have seen many people relapse, and even die, over mismanaging their pain medication. Frequently the relapse starts with an acute pain episode such as dental work that requires pain medication. Some people experience problems when they develop a chronic pain condition that does not respond to non-narcotic interventions. In either case, the person failed to develop an effective medication management plan.

Managing pain medication is an issue that people dealing with chronic pain may face at some point in their recovery journey. Yet most people don't know how to develop an effective plan of action. When you are in recovery for chemical dependency—whether the substance is prescription drugs, alcohol, marijuana, etc.—the risk of relapse is always present. It's unrealistic to expect that you will never have a medical or dental situation where pain management is needed. And if you also have a chronic pain condition, relapse prevention becomes even more crucial.

> ## Two Major Pain Management Roadblocks
> • Overmedicating Pain
> • Undermedicating Pain

There are two major problems when you are in recovery and experiencing a pain condition that requires medication—*overmedicating* and *undermedicating*. Even an acute pain condition such as dental pain may lead to relapse problems. When overmedicated you can develop substance-induced problems or even addiction. When you are undermedicated, you may decide to use self-defeating behaviors such as alcohol, other drug use, or even suicide to cope with your pain. I devote a significant section of chapter nine to help you develop a plan for managing pain medication in recovery.

Looking at the Solution
Knowledge Is Power

To effectively manage a pain condition it's very important that you understand exactly what is going on with your body. When in pain, you experience both physical and psychological symptoms. To understand the language of pain, you must learn to listen to how the pain echoes and reverberates between the physical, psychological, and social dimensions of your human condition. Pain is truly a total human experience that affects all aspects of human functioning.

> To understand the language of pain we need to listen to its echoes among the physical, psychological, and social dimensions of our humanity.

When you're in pain for a long period of time, you can feel victimized by your pain. You may hate your pain. You may want to escape from your pain. You may even become willing to do anything to get relief. Unfortunately, many people get that relief by using self-defeating behaviors, including the abuse of pain medication.

> You will manage your pain better when you are proactive in your own treatment and recovery process.

The research on recovery from chronic pain is clear. You're most likely to successfully manage your pain by becoming actively involved in your own treatment. Your chances of success go up as you start learning as much as possible about your pain and effective pain management. The next chapter will help you do this by explaining the *Addiction Pain Syn-*

drome and the biopsychosocial nature of pain. Future chapters will describe an effective *Addiction-Free Pain Management* (APM) protocol and show you how two of my patients, Donna and Matt, used the APM process of recovery.

Knowledge is power. Once you know what is really going on with your body and mind you can start to take action to effectively manage your pain. In fact, you need to stop believing pain is your enemy and begin to embrace it as your friend. I know this is easier said than done. Many of my patients have looked at me like I'm crazy when I tell them they must make peace with their pain and that pain is their friend. They tell me—very strongly—that they can't buy it, but nevertheless it is true.

> Make peace with your pain.
> Stop believing pain is your enemy.
> Begin embracing pain as your friend.

As you will see in the next chapter, pain sensations are essential for human survival. Without pain you would have no way of knowing that something is wrong with your body. So without pain you would be unable to take action to correct the problem or situation that is causing the condition. However, with chronic pain management it is crucial that you choose the correct type of action or you could end up in the trap of addiction.

Coping with Anticipatory Pain

When you're in chronic pain you hurt. Doing certain *things* can make you hurt worse. So you come to believe that these things will *"always cause me to hurt."* In other words, you associate those things with pain. You believe that every time you do those things, you'll have pain. Because you believe you're going to hurt, you can activate the physiological pain system just by thinking about doing something that you believe will cause you to hurt. This is called **anticipatory pain**. You anticipate that something will make you hurt. That, in turn, activates your physiological pain system. This makes you start hurting even before you begin doing whatever it is that you believe will cause you to hurt. All you have to do is to start thinking about doing that *thing*.

Once the physical pain system is activated, the anticipatory pain reaction can actually make your pain symptoms worse. Whenever you feel the pain, you *interpret it* in a way that makes it worse. You *start thinking* about the pain in a way that makes it worse. You *tell yourself* that the pain is "awful and terrible," and that "I can't handle the pain." You *convince yourself* it's hopeless, you'll always hurt, and there's nothing you can do about it. This way of thinking causes you to develop emotional reactions that further intensify the pain response. The increased perception of pain causes you to keep changing your behavior in ways that create even more unnecessary limitations and more emotional discomfort. This can make you feel trapped in a progressive cycle of disability.

> ## This is horrible, awful, terrible!

Your expectations—what you believe it will be like when you experience pain—affect your brain chemistry. Your brain chemistry can either intensify or reduce the amount of physical pain that you experience. What you think and how you manage your feelings in anticipation of feeling pain can make the pain either more severe or less severe. In other words, you'll usually get the level of pain and dysfunction that you expect—a self-fulfilling prophecy.

> ## You'll usually get the level of pain and dysfunction that you expect!

The anticipation of an expected pain level can influence the degree to which you experience pain. When your self-talk is saying, "This is horrible, awful, terrible," the brain tends to amplify the pain signal. When this occurs, your level of distress increases—you suffer, remaining a victim to your pain.

But you can learn how to change your anticipatory response to pain. You can lower the amount of pain that you anticipate by changing what you believe will happen when you start to hurt. You can also change your thinking—your self-talk—and how you manage your emotions. You can learn new ways of responding to old situations that can cause pain. As you come to believe that you can really do things that will make the pain reaction bearable and manageable, your brain responds by influencing special neurons that reduce the intensity of the pain. Your brain becomes less responsive to an incoming pain signal.

There are things you can do that will make you habitually less responsive to incoming pain signals. Herein lies the rationale for biofeedback, positive self-talk, and meditation as pain control methods. In any event, both ascending (pain signals coming from the point of injury to the brain) and descending nerve pathways (signals from the brain to the point of injury) will influence or modify the effects of pain on your body. I cover this further in the next chapter when you look at the *pain system* and *pain versus suffering.*

There Are No Magic Fixes

It's important to remember that the treatment for chronic pain does not include magical interventions or quick fixes; rather, effective treatment is a combination of proven psychological approaches in addition to medication management and other non-pharmacological, or *holistic* interventions that address all the issues people in chronic pain experience. The three core components of APM are based on an accurate understanding of the *Addiction Pain Syndrome.* Knowledge about the addiction pain syndrome is your most powerful tool in recovery. So what is the Addiction Pain Syndrome? Let's go to the next chapter to find out.

Chapter Two

The Addiction Pain Syndrome

Understanding Pain and Addiction

Addiction-Free Pain Management (APM) is a system that can help you to manage your chronic pain without abusing or becoming addicted to pain medication. To fully understand APM, you need to understand the Addiction Pain Syndrome, which is composed of three parts: (1) addiction, (2) pain, and (3) the pain system.

Understanding Addiction

I will be using the term "addiction" to discuss what the *Diagnostic and Statistic Manual of Mental Disorders, 4th Edition* (DSM-IV) classifies as "substance use disorders" and others refer to as "chemical dependency." In this book I will use the following definition of addiction: **Addiction is a collection of symptoms (i.e., a syndrome) that is caused by a negative response to taking mood-altering substances and has ten major characteristics**. I want to point out here that there is a difference between addiction and physical dependence, which I will cover a little later in this chapter.

The characteristics of addiction are shown in the table, followed by a brief explanation of each characteristic.

Addictive Disorder Symptoms	
1. Euphoria	6. Inability to Abstain
2. Craving	7. Addiction-Centered Lifestyle
3. Tolerance	8. Addictive Lifestyle Losses
4. Loss of Control	9. Continued Use Despite Problems
5. Withdrawal	10. Substance-Induced Organic Mental Disorders

Let's look at each of these characteristics in a little more detail.

Euphoria

People use drugs because they work—they change how you think or feel. This is true of pain medications and other potential drugs of abuse including alcohol. If you experience a unique sense of well-being when you use medication or another drug, you are at high risk of becoming addicted to that drug.

```
┌─────────────────────────────────────────────────┐
│          Positive Reinforcement for Use          │
└─────────────────────────────────────────────────┘
```

Recent research shows that when you are genetically susceptible to being addicted to a specific drug, your brain will release large amounts of brain reward chemicals whenever that drug is used. It's this high level of brain reward chemicals that cause the unique feeling of well-being that many people who become addicted experience when using their drug of choice (including prescription medication). In this book I call this unique feeling of well-being **euphoria**.

```
┌─────────────────────────────────────────────────┐
│            Euphoria vs. Intoxication             │
└─────────────────────────────────────────────────┘
```

It's important to distinguish between euphoria (the unique sense of well-being experienced when using a drug of choice) and intoxication (the symptoms of dysfunction that occur when a person's use exceeds the limits of their tolerance to a drug). Addicts do not use their drug of choice to get intoxicated and become dysfunctional. The opposite is true. People who are addicted use their drug of choice to feel good and experience a unique feeling of well-being that will allow them to function better.

You can become addicted to this state of euphoria wherein you crave this unique sense of well-being, and feel empty or incomplete when you can't feel this way. You feel deprived when you can't experience it again. You may even experience deprivation anxiety, which is a fear that if you can't get your drug of choice (i.e., you're deprived of it), you won't be able to feel good or to function normally.

> ## Positive reinforcement leads to cravings.

Positive reinforcement is biopsychosocial in nature. Biologically the drug of choice causes a release of pleasure chemicals that create a unique sense of well-being. Psychologically, "I come to believe the drug is good for me because it makes me feel good in the moment." This is called emotional reasoning ("If it feels good it must be good for me"). You then begin adjusting your social network to accommodate these beliefs: "Anyone who supports my use of my drug of choice is my friend. Anyone who challenges the use of my drug of choice is my enemy." The result is the development of a drug-centered lifestyle.

The stronger the positive reinforcement that is experienced when you use your drug of choice, the greater the risk that you will become addicted. This is because strong biological reinforcement from drug use creates a craving cycle.

Craving

Addiction starts when you receive a reward, payoff, or gratification from taking a drug. This reward may be the relief of pain or the creation of a feeling of euphoria. You continue to use the drug because it provides a quick positive reward.

With a pattern of consistent drug use you come to rely on the drug to provide this reward. This leads to addiction, which is also called chemical dependency. You need to use the drug to successfully accomplish one or more life tasks. Once you become addicted, you experience psychological distress when the substance you are addicted to is removed. So when you become addicted to a drug for relief or euphoria, you experience anxiety when the drug is no longer available. Albert Ellis calls this **deprivation anxiety**. You're anxious because you have been deprived of a drug that you believe you need in order to function normally.

> ## Deprivation anxiety leads to obsession.

The deprivation anxiety then causes you to start thinking about the drug. *Obsession* is out-of-control thinking about the reward that could be achieved by using the substance. Obsession can lead to *compulsion*—the irrational desire for the drug. Obsession and compulsion combine together to create a powerful *craving,* or feeling a need for the drug.

> ## Obsession + Compulsion = Craving

This cycle of obsession, compulsion, and craving creates a strong urge or pressure to seek out and use the drug even if you consciously know that it's not in your best interest to do so. Over time this reward continues to be reinforced, leading to an increased need for the drug. This leads to tolerance.

Tolerance

There is a biological component to developing tolerance. The increased need for the drug leads to drug-seeking behavior. There are also psychological and social components to this developmental process.

On the biological level, after drug-seeking behavior has been established, the brain undergoes certain adaptive changes to continue functioning despite the presence of the drug—your brain chemistry actually changes. This adaptation is called **tolerance.**

Psychologically you start believing that you need the drug. When you start to experience difficulty obtaining enough of the drug, you start feeling anxious and afraid. Socially you begin to experience difficulty with other people because of the time and energy you are expending.

Loss of Control

The final stage of the craving cycle and development of tolerance is a loss of control over your drug use. You begin to develop an even higher tolerance for the drug. In other words, it takes more of the drug to get the same effect. If you keep using the same amount of the drug, you experience less of an effect. So you begin using more of the drug or seeking out stronger drugs that will give the same reinforcing effect.

At times the drug is taken in such large quantities that you become intoxicated or dysfunctional. This dysfunction creates life problems. At this point, if you stop using the drug, you will experience uncomfortable physical and emotional problems. This leads to lowered motivation to stop the drug use.

Withdrawal

Withdrawal is marked by the development of a specific withdrawal syndrome upon the cessation of use. In some cases you may use the same or similar drug to relieve or avoid the withdrawal syndrome.

> ## Withdrawal as Negative Reinforcement
> ## (i.e. Anguish or Dysphoria)

Once tolerance and loss of control take place, further abnormalities occur in the brain when drugs are removed. In other words, the brain loses its capacity to function normally when drugs are not present. This leads to low-grade abstinence-based brain dysfunction, which is distinct and different from acute withdrawal. This brain dysfunction is marked by feelings of discomfort, increased cravings, and difficulty finding gratification from other behaviors. You don't like how this feels: it's unpleasant, it's uncomfortable, and it's painful.

You want to avoid pain. You want to feel good. This desire to avoid pain causes what is called **negative reinforcement**. Whenever you do something that makes you feel bad, you get negatively reinforced. In other words, your brain reaction conditions you to avoid the pain by avoiding whatever it is that causes the pain. If abstinence causes pain and using chemicals causes pleasure, you get conditioned to seek out medication or alcohol and other drugs. You also tend to avoid situations where you need to be abstinent.

> ## Euphoria + Craving + Tolerance = Biological Reinforcement
>
> - People who experience biological reinforcement are more likely to use drugs regularly and heavily.
>
> - People who use drugs regularly and heavily are more likely to develop an addictive disorder.

Inability to Abstain

As a result of your experiences created by the biological reinforcement and high tolerance, you come to believe that your drug of choice is good for you and will magically fix you or make you better. You start to develop an addictive belief system. You come to view people who support your drug use as friends and want to avoid people who fail to support it.

> ## Addictive Beliefs

At this point you're experiencing both positive and negative reinforcement to keep using. If you continue to use you experience euphoria and pain relief. This occurs because the brain releases large amounts of *reward chemicals* when you use your drug of choice.

If you stop using, you experience dysphoria or pain and suffering. You start to experience a sense of a low-grade agitated depression and the inability to experience pleasure. You begin to believe that you have no choice but to keep using.

Addiction-Centered Lifestyle

You may attract and are attracted to other individuals who share strong positive attitudes toward your continued use of drugs (problematic pain medication). By this time you usually have an enabling support system that condones and encourages your continued use. You become immersed in an addiction-centered system.

A Pattern of Heavy and Regular Use

Addictive Lifestyle Losses

You begin to create distance from others who support sobriety (appropriate use of your medication) and surround yourself with people who support ongoing problematic chemical use. The pattern of biological reinforcement has motivated you to build a belief system and lifestyle that supports heavy and regular use.

You are now in a position where you will voluntarily use larger amounts of medication (or other drugs including alcohol) with greater frequency until progressive addiction and the accompanying physical, psychological, and social problems occur. Your life eventually becomes unbearable and unmanageable. You start experiencing a downward spiral of serious problems.

Continued Use Despite Problems

Unfortunately, this downward spiral leads to continued drug use in spite of the negative consequences. This inability to control drug use causes problems. The problems cause pain. The pain activates a craving. The craving drives you to start using the drug to get the relief that you believe you need—*and deserve.*

As a result, when you're addicted and experience adverse consequences from your addiction, the adverse consequences cause cravings instead of correction. You keep using drugs to gain the immediate reward or relief despite the progressively more serious life problems.

Substance-Induced Organic Mental Disorders

The progressive damage of psychoactive chemicals on the brain creates growing problems with judgment and impulse control. As a result, your behavior begins to spiral out of control. Your cognitive capacities needed to think abstractly about the problem have also been impaired, and you are now locked into a pattern marked by denial and circular systems of reasoning.

> ## Progressive neurological and neuropsychological impairments lead to denial.

You are unable to recognize the pattern of problems related to the use of your medication or alcohol and other drugs. When you experience problems and are challenged by them, you begin to experience physical, psychological, and social deterioration. Unless you develop an unexpected insight or are confronted by serious problems or people in your life, your progressive problems are likely to continue until serious damage results.

> ## Chemical Dependency vs. Addiction

It's important to note here that not everyone who uses pain medication on an ongoing basis will become addicted. You may, in fact, become physically dependent to the medication but may not experience the addiction cycle covered above. In a later chapter I will discuss the *Recovery and Relapse Indicators* for those of you who need to take psychoactive medication on a continuing basis.

Now that you have a better understanding of addictive disorders, you also need to learn more about your pain and the biopsychosocial processes that influence it. This is important in order to gain the most benefit from the APM recovery process.

Understanding Pain Disorders

An Overview of the Biopsychosocial Components of Pain
In order to understand pain management you need to first understand the concept of pain. Pain is a signal from the body to the brain that tells you something is wrong. There are three components of pain: biological, psychological, and social/cultural.

> Pain is a signal from the body to the brain
> that tells you something is wrong.

Pain is a total biopsychosocial experience. You hurt physically. You psychologically respond to the pain by thinking, feeling, and acting. You think about the pain and try to figure out what is causing it and why you're hurting. You experience emotional reactions to the pain. You may get angry, frightened, or frustrated by your pain. You talk about your pain with family, friends, and coworkers who help you to develop a social and cultural context for assigning meaning to your personal pain experience and taking appropriate action.

> ## Three Levels of Pain Management

Modern pain management systematically approaches the treatment of pain at all three levels simultaneously. This means using physical treatments to reduce the intensity of your physical pain. It also means using psychological treatments to identify and change your thoughts, feelings, and behaviors that are making your pain more intense and replacing them with positive thinking, as well as feeling and behavior management skills that can reduce the intensity of your pain.

Finally, effective pain management must involve not only you, but also the significant people in your life who can help you to develop a social and cultural context in which to experience your pain in a way that will reduce suffering.

> ## The Three Components of Pain
> - Biological
> - Psychological
> - Social/Cultural

Biological pain is a signal that something is going wrong with your body. **Psychological Pain** results from the meaning that you assign to the pain signal. **Social and Cultural Pain,** also known as suffering, results from the *social and cultural meaning* assigned by other people to the pain that is being experienced, and whether or not the pain is recognized as being severe enough to warrant a socially approved *sick* role.

These three components determine whether the signal from your body to your brain is interpreted as pain or suffering. I'll discuss more about pain signals and the pain system later in this chapter.

Pain vs. Suffering

The psychological meaning that you assign to the physical pain signal will determine whether you simply feel pain ("Ouch, this hurts!") or experience suffering ("Because I hurt, something awful or terrible is happening!"). Although pain and suffering are often used interchangeably, there is an important distinction that needs to be made. Pain is an unpleasant signal telling you that something is wrong with your body. Suffering results from the meaning or interpretation your brain assigns to the pain.

Pain Is Biopsychosocial

• **Biological Pain:** a signal that something is going wrong with your body

• **Psychological Pain:** the meaning that you assign to the pain signal

• **Social/Cultural Pain:** the societally approved "sick" role assigned to you concerning your pain

---

Many people irrationally believe the following: "I shouldn't have pain!" or "Because I have pain and I'm having trouble managing the pain, there must be something wrong with me." A big step toward pain management occurs when you can reduce your level of suffering by identifying and changing your irratlonal beliefs about your pain, which in turn decreases your stress and overall suffering.

Because of the two parts—pain and suffering—pain management must also have two components: physical and psychological. The way you sense or experience pain—its intensity and duration—will affect how well you are able to manage it. In addition, there are two major classifications of pain that need clarification: aoute pain and chronic pain.

Acute Pain and Chronic Pain

It is important to understand the difference between acute pain and chronic pain, especially when there is a need to manage the pain with potentially addictive medication.

Acute pain tells your body that something has gone wrong or that damage to the system has occurred. The source of the pain can usually be easily identified, and typically does not last very long. An example of acute pain is when you touch a hot burner on the stove.

A **chronic pain** condition will linger long after the initial injury, sometimes for years. In many cases chronic pain no longer serves a useful purpose. To be considered a chronic pain condition, the symptoms will have a duration of at least six months. Some examples of chronic pain are ongoing back pain or frequent cluster headaches.

> **Acute Pain** is short lived.
> **Chronic Pain** lasts six months or more.

Effective pain management requires accurate identification of the physical and psychological components of the pain disorder. This is where the *Addiction-Free Pain Management Workbook* should be used. As you will see in chapter five, there is a way to determine whether your pain condition is more physiological or psychological.

Historically, addictive disorders and pain disorders have been treated as separate issues. In the next chapter I will demonstrate that to effectively implement Addiction-Free Pain

Management, both the addictive disorder and the pain disorder must be adequately addressed at the same time. In addition, the physical, psychological, and social implications of these disorders must also be dealt with.

> **Addressing both the pain disorder and the addictive disorder is crucial.**

The Neurophysiology of Pain

As I discussed earlier, pain is a complex combination of biopsychosocial phenomena. In this section I refer to the work of Dr. Mark Stanford to look at the neurophysiology of pain.

Let's start by examining the word "neurophysiology." The root "neuro" refers to the nerves or more precisely how the actions of the brain and nerves are involved in the pain response. The word "physiology" refers to the physical aspects of pain, or more precisely, how the total human organism responds and adapts to pain.

This section will give you an accurate yet easy-to-understand model for explaining the complex biopsychosocial symptoms that you experience. It will also prepare you to understand why many of the treatment methodologies described later in this book are both effective and necessary.

Despite my efforts to simplify this section, the information I am trying to explain is rather complex. My goal is not to describe the technical details of pain neurophysiology but to present some basic theories and concepts, which form the basis of current pain management approaches.

Pain as a Signal that Communicates Information

The easiest way to understand pain is to recognize that every time you feel pain your body is attempting to tell you that something is wrong. Pain sensations are critical to human survival. Without pain you would have no way of knowing that something is wrong with your body. So without pain you would be unable to take action to correct the problem or situation that is causing your pain.

What is your pain trying to tell you?

Whenever you are experiencing pain, it's always helpful to ask, "What is my pain trying to tell me?" The pain is trying to tell you that something is wrong and that you had better find out what exactly is wrong and find a way to fix it.

To understand the language of pain, you must learn to understand how the pain echoes and reverberates between the physical, psychological, and social dimensions of the human condition. Pain is truly a total human experience that affects all aspects of human functioning.

Understanding the Pain System

Every human being has a pain system that has a combination of pain receptors and pain circuits. As you continue, it may be useful to refer to the Pain System Diagram (see page 42). This diagram shows some of the pain receptor sites and pain circuits that comprise the human pain system.

You also have specialized and general pain receptors and circuits. These receptors and circuits usually function very well, alerting you when something is wrong.

- **Pain receptors are nerve cells that detect when something is wrong.**

- **Pain circuits are a series of nerve cells that transmit the message to your brain that something is wrong.**

- **Pain is the signal or warning that indicates something is wrong.**

Physically, the experience of pain originates in receptors that are located throughout the body. Some of these receptors are located deep within the body, providing sensations about muscle aches, pulled tendons, and fluid-filled, swollen joints.

Other receptors, such as in the skin, provide pain sensations when cuts, burns, or abrasions have occurred near the surface of the body. Many times the skin receptors respond to the signal generated from the localized damage to tissue. For example, a skin cut will essentially cause various cells to produce and release a variety of chemical messengers that stimulate pain receptors into action from the area of injury.

Pain System Diagram

**Ascending
and Descending
Pain Circuits**

**Pain
Receptor Sites**

Pain Receptors and Circuits

The human brain and nervous system have **pain recep-tors,** which respond to the pain where it occurs in the body. There are also **pain circuits** (sometimes these circuits are called *neuropathways*) that transmit pain signals from the local site of the pain to the spinal cord and then to the brain itself. As the pain signal moves along its primary circuit or pathway, other secondary pain neurons are activated creating a wide variety of different types of pain signals.

Some of these signals simply report the presence of pain ("I hurt" or "I don't hurt"). Other signals report the intensity of the pain ("I hurt a little" or "I hurt a lot"). Still other pain signals report the location of the pain ("My stomach hurts") and whether the pain is associated with an internal or external injury ("My stomach hurts deep in my gut" or "The skin on my stomach hurts"). Other pain signals report the type of pain ("My pain burns or it throbs").

All of these different pain signals are transmitted into the spinal cord through nerve pathways. The nerve pathways transmit the pain signal information to other specialized pain neurons, which in turn send the information to different areas of the brain.

Certain types of pain will activate an *automatic protective reflex* (you suddenly pull your hand away from the hot handle of a frying pan without thinking about it). Other types of pain burst into conscious awareness prompting you to try and figure out what is wrong.

Specialized and General Purpose Pain Receptors and Circuits

The human body has **specialty pain receptors and circuits** that are dedicated exclusively to recognizing and transmitting information about pain. There are, for example, separate pain receptors and circuits that respond to skin cuts. This provides you with the ability to recognize and respond to certain types of pain quickly.

You also have **general purpose receptors and circuits** that are capable of detecting and transmitting pain signals and other sensations that give information about other physiological processes.

- Specialty Pain Receptors and Circuits
- General Purpose Receptors and Circuits

Because pain is an indication of threat or emergency, these general purpose receptors and circuits give your pain signals top priority. When an emergency pain signal competes with other routine non-emergency sensations, the routine sensations are temporarily shut down or distorted so the transmission of the pain signal can be given a top priority.

As a result, there can be a **generalized nonspecific response** to pain signals. In other words pain signals can disrupt other systems of your body that are not directly affected by the injury or illness causing the pain. This occurs by disrupting the routine flow of sensation.

Pain and the Cascade Effect

As you can see, the process of experiencing pain is complex and has the potential of affecting all areas of your brain and body. When your pain is intense and prolonged, there is a widespread **cascade effect** that results in an extensive disruption in your normal functioning.

To understand this cascade effect let's look at what happens when you accidentally cut your hand with a sharp piece of glass. The cut activates specific pain receptors, which in turn begin sending pain signals down a pain circuit or pathway. As the signal moves along the pain circuit, a variety of signals related to the pain are activated. These signals are transmitted through the spinal chord to your brain. One part of your brain's cortex receives the information about the sudden pain that has just happened. Another part determines where your body has been hurt. Another part determines what type of pain you are experiencing, and still another part determines how severe (intense) your pain is.

The Immediate Reflex Response

While the various parts of the brain are communicating about your pain, another part of the nervous system activates an immediate reflex response. This reflex causes a quick withdrawal from the point of the pain-producing situation (in this case the piece of glass).

The rapid behavioral withdrawal reflex is a response that is based largely in your spinal cord and less so in your brain. Other areas within your brain begin activating the autonomic nervous system that, among other things, increases heart rate and still another part of the brain signals the hypothalamus to start secreting a cascade of chemical reactions.

Meanwhile, your brain overrides a number of routine neurological circuits and reroutes available body resources to respond to the pain. You quickly enter into a high stress response that prepares you to fight, freeze, or flee from the danger.

This cascade of effects from the original pain sensation occurs on many levels and involves a variety of different areas within your nervous system. As a result a wide variety of nervous system chemicals are produced and dumped into your blood while other brain chemicals are rapidly absorbed or depleted. Pain doesn't just hurt. It changes your most basic neurophysiological processes.

Anticipation of Pain Affects How Pain Is Experienced

The anticipation of an expected pain level can influence the degree to which you experience your pain. In some cases, when your anticipatory level of pain expectation is lowered, your brain responds by influencing special neurons. As you saw in the last chapter this renders your brain less responsive to an incoming pain signal and your sensation of pain decreases. Herein lies the rationale for biofeedback and meditation as pain control methods. In any event, both ascending (pain signals coming from the point of injury to the brain) and descending nerve pathways (signals from the brain to the point of injury) will influence or modify the effects on your body.

The Pain Spiral

You can begin a downward spiral when a *cascade effect* occurs and is coupled with a negative *anticipation effect*. You begin to think like a victim. You start feeling hopeless and helpless, which often leads to grief and depression.

This condition is covered in another chapter, but for now it's important to remember that the cumulative biopsychosocial effects of chronic pain lead to this pain spiral. When you try to cope with this condition by using addictive medications, the downward addiction spiral is intensified. In addition, your brain is attempting to adapt by telling other parts of your body to produce additional chemicals as it tries to manage the situation.

While it is important to realize that most of the time your pain tells you there is something wrong with your body and is part of your defense system, the fact that pain may not always be serving a useful purpose is sometimes not as obvious.

Impaired Pain System Leads to Chronic Pain

As with any sensory system, pain receptors and circuits can become impaired, resulting in chronic pain that cannot be attributed to any identified physical problem. Probably the greatest challenge in regard to understanding the biological aspects of pain is why it sometimes continues even after a painful stimulus has been removed. To help clarify pain further it's necessary to briefly describe three types of pain.

Three Types of Pain

Pain can be organized into different categories depending on the type of pain. The experience of pain, regardless of the pain-producing source, has the single physical feature of discomfort. However, there are actually three types of pain.

- Type One: Direct Pain
- Type Two: Indirect Pain
- Type Three: Systemic Pain

Type One Pain is directly related to a pain source. This type of pain is well known and easily understood. There is a direct cause-and-effect relationship between the pain source and the sensation of painful stimulation. Examples of type one pain include burns, abrasions, cuts, and so on.

Type Two Pain is indirectly related to a pain source. This type of pain includes the pain of inflammation; such as in a sprained ankle or swollen knee, where there is swelling, redness, and the skin is hot to the touch around the affected area. These two types of pain and their treatments are well understood by the medical community and usually treated effectively.

Type Three Pain is not related to a pain source and is systemic or universal in nature. Type three pain still remains somewhat of a mystery to the medical and scientific communities. This type of pain does not possess the clear and distinct cause-effect relationship between the source of pain and pain sensation.

Chronic Pain Is Often Type Three Pain

Type three pain includes the condition of neuropathy. This is a condition where the pain nerve receptors and circuitry are supersensitive and interpret ordinary input to the brain as painful sensations. It's like putting an electrical signal through an unnecessary amplifier and the high voltage burns out or damages the appliance.

Because there is no pain source, per se, for type three pain, surgery is not a useful intervention, and alternative treatment methods need to be considered. Chronic pain is often a result of the pain signal getting turned on but unable to get turned off.

Unanswered Questions

While the physiology of pain can be explained to a large extent, this sensory experience is a very complex phenomenon. There are still many unanswered questions about the various types of pain sensation.

For example, many of you have experienced the muscle aches and pain after a full day of strenuous physical work, such as in a backyard garden. Your muscles can get tight, sore, and aching due to excess use, lifting, digging, and stretching. However, if you apply some light massage or bodywork to this type of pain the intensity of your pain decreases and sometimes disappears altogether. This example seems initially contradictory in that if your muscles are aching, you might think that the last thing to help alleviate the pain would be to apply pressure through bodywork.

On the other hand, pain sensation will also result when a sensory experience is pushed to the extreme. That is, when the pain receptor limit is reached and surpassed, sensory experience can change from pleasant to painful. An example is when heat receptors in the skin are stimulated by warm sunlight. The results are usually experienced as pleasurable sensations. However, these same receptors also signal a painful sensation if overstimulated (pushed passed a certain threshold) such as in the case of severe sunburn.

Understanding the Addiction Pain Syndrome

Pulling It All Together

Your final task in this chapter is to understand the connection between pain and addiction. Pain is the reason you may start using potentially addictive substances. Chronic use of psychoactive medication plus genetic susceptibility can lead from pain relief to increased tolerance. Eventually the addictive substance no longer manages your pain symptoms. In fact, it often increases or amplifies the pain signals—the pain-rebound effect. The end result is severe biopsychosocial pain and problems.

Historically, pain disorders and addictive disorders have been treated as separate issues. Pain clinics have had great success in treating chronic pain conditions. Chemical dependency treatment centers have had success in treating addictive disorders. However, both modalities struggle when the patient is suffering with both conditions.

As you can see from the Addiction Pain Syndrome diagram (see page 50), chemical dependency recovery or treatment programs cover about a third of the problem (the *addictive disorder zone*) when dealing with a chronic pain patient. The pain clinics cover a different third of the problem (the *pain disorder zone*). Each of the above modalities misses about two thirds of the problem.

Sometimes chemical dependency treatment centers recognize the need to refer a patient to a pain specialist or the pain clinics refer a patient to a chemical dependency specialist. This is definitely an improvement. Now about two thirds of the patient's needs are being addressed (both the addictive disorder zone and the pain disorder zone). But what about the third zone?

The center area of the diagram is the *addiction pain syndrome zone*. This is why I developed the Addiction-Free Pain Management (APM) System that is described in the next chapter. APM addresses all three areas: The addictive disorder zone, the pain disorder zone, and the addiction pain syndrome zone.

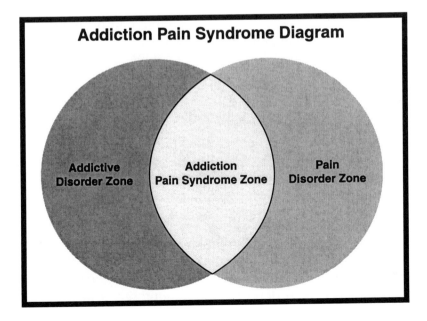

Synergistic Symptoms

When addictive disorders and pain disorders coexist, the negative impact more than doubles. Addictive disorders lead to one set of biopsychosocial problems, and the pain disorders lead to another set of problems. Now 1 + 1 no longer equals 2; rather 1 + 1 equals 3 or more. This is called synergism. **Synergism** is a condition where the combined action is greater in total effect than the sum of the parts.

Take another look at the Addiction Pain Syndrome Diagram and notice the area labeled the addictive disorder zone. Now look at the pain disorder zone. When these two zones are added together you can see the sum of both zones and a new zone—the addiction pain sndrome zone. New symptoms occur due to the combined effect.

Synergistic Treatment System

The APM system uses three types of components to treat the synergistic symptoms, which include all three of the addiction pain syndrome zones. The first treatment component uses the eight **core clinical processes**, which are the foundation of the *Addiction-Free Pain Management Workbook.* Second are the **medication management components**, and third are the **holistic treatment processes**. I fully explain these three APM components in the next chapter.

The Synergistic Treatment System

- Core Clinical Processes
- Medication Management Components
- Holistic Treatment Processes

Developing an effective treatment plan also depends on knowing which stage of the problem you are in. If you have been abusing your medication it's important to understand which stage of the addiction process you are at and how much damage has been done by your inappropriate use of pain medication. As you move into recovery, it's essential to understand which stage of the developmental process of recovery you are in.

In the following chapter I am going to describe *The Developmental Model of Recovery* and *Addiction-Free Pain Management.* I will show you how the APM System effectively addresses an addictive disorder and a pain disorder at the same time.

Chapter Three

The Addiction-Free Pain Management System

The Developmental Model of Recovery

Once the progression of addiction has been halted the next step is to determine what stage of the recovery process you're in. This is where an understanding of the CENAPS® Developmental Model of Recovery is very important. I'm going to present a brief overview here. If you want to explore this model further please refer to *Passages Through Recovery* by Terence T. Gorski.

The Gorski-CENAPS® Developmental Model of Recovery is based on the premise that addiction and its related mental and personality disorders are chronic lifestyle related conditions that require a long-term developmental process of recovery. This model is similar to the research models developed by Stephanie Brown or James Prochaska and Carlo DiClemente. The CENAPS® developmental recovery process is conceptualized as moving through a series of six stages.

The Six Stages of Recovery

- Stage Zero: Active Addiction
- Stage One: Transition
- Stage Two: Stabilization
- Stage Three: Early Recovery
- Stage Four: Middle Recovery
- Stage Five: Late Recovery
- Stage Six: Maintenance

Stage Zero

Before you get to the first stage you're in **stage zero** (also known as pre-treatment or pre-contemplation). During this stage you're actively abusing your pain medication, receiving substantial *perceived* benefits from your use, experiencing few *perceived* adverse consequences, and as a result you see no reason to seek help. It usually takes some type of motivational crisis (medical problem, family problem, job problem, etc.) to halt this cycle.

Transition

During the **transition stage** (also known as contemplation) the primary focus is on interrupting denial and treatment resistance. If you are in this stage you're usually experiencing a motivating crisis, coupled with a failure of your usual coping tools (i.e., your pain medication no longer works like you want it to). The primary task is to help you recognize and accept the need for treatment.

Stabilization

During the **stabilization stage** the primary focus is breaking the addiction cycle, managing withdrawal, stabilizing mental status (thinking and feelings), and managing situational life crisis. If you are addicted and have chronic pain, this stage requires that you develop safer pain management tools while developing hope—which is moving from victim to empowerment.

Early Recovery

During the **early recovery stage** the primary focus is learning about your addictive disorder and pain disorder, as well as any related mental and personality disorders. You need to learn about the recovery process, to establish a structured recovery program, and to integrate basic skills for identifying and managing addictive thoughts, feelings, and behaviors.

Middle Recovery

During the **middle recovery stage** the primary focus is on repairing damage caused by your addiction to significant others, to your work, social, intimate, and friendship systems. Middle recovery is also the time for you to fully resolve the grief and loss issues caused by your pain disorder and/or your addictive disorder. It's a time to establish a balanced lifestyle, as well as developing an effective pain management and recovery program.

Late Recovery

During the **late recovery stage** the focus is to help you make changes in self-defeating personality styles and self-destructive lifestyle structures that interfere with maintaining sobriety, effective pain management, and responsibility. Because many people with chronic pain disorders have also experienced past physical and/or emotional trauma, those issues need to be processed and resolved.

Maintenance

During the **maintenance stage** the primary focus is on the continuance of sobriety, effective pain management, and responsibility. In this stage you are learning how to obtain a better quality of life while actively participating in your developmental life process.

Understanding and implementing the developmental model of recovery is crucial for helping you recover from the Addiction Pain Syndrome.

> ## APM is the concurrent treatment of pain and addictive disorders.

In the previous chapter you saw how addictive disorders and pain disorders interact—*the Addiction Pain Syndrome.* Now that you understand how these two conditions overlap, I'll use the remainder of this chapter to define and explain the overlapping treatment system—*Addiction-Free Pain Management.*

Addiction-Free Pain Management Defined

First of all, let's look at the term "addiction-free." To understand this term, you need to recognize the difference between addiction and dependency. You also need to remember the earlier definition of the addictive disorder, which includes biological rewards, craving cycle, loss of control, and negative consequences.

Many chronic pain patients are biologically dependent on their medication. In other words their body and brain physically need the medication, but they *do not* exhibit the addictive biopsychosocial tendencies described in the first chapter—this combination is called physical dependency. To be considered addiction-free you must be free of *inappropriate* psychoactive chemicals (no addictive tendencies) and you're using other non-pharmacological treatment modalities to manage your pain, such as the ones described later in this chapter.

In some instances "addiction-free" may mean that if you must take mood-altering medication, you are able to do so exactly as prescribed. You use the medication for pain relief but *do not* use the medication to achieve a state of euphoria or mood alteration. You don't obsess about your medication, or become compulsive about taking it, and you *do not* experience negative consequences from using it. This is a fairly simple description of addiction-free pain management, which I will expand upon as you move further into this book.

> Addiction-Free Pain Management (APM) is the ability to manage a chronic pain condition without experiencing the negative consequences of addiction.

The Development of Addiction-Free Pain Management

Now that we have common definitions of addiction and addiction-free pain management, we're ready to look at the developmental process of the APM system. I will do this by explaining the five developmental stages that APM has undergone over the past two decades. It's important to remember that this system is still a "work in progress" and by reading this book you become a part of its evolution.

APM Stage One: A Personal Recovery Experience

APM Stage Two: Working with Chronic Pain Patients

APM Stage Three: Applying the CENAPS® Model

APM Stage Four: Field-testing the System

APM Stage Five: Spreading the Word

APM Stage One:
Pain Management—A Personal Recovery Experience

The first seeds for Addiction-Free Pain Management (APM) were actually planted in 1962, but they did not really develop until nearly twenty years later. The conception and initial foundation were the result of looking back on an elementary school accident and the narcotic pain medication I received. That one incident caused many problems that continued throughout my adolescence and early adult life from repeated exposure to pain medication.

The developmental process or evolution began when I experienced a workplace accident in the early 1980s and finally realized that I wanted to live my life free of narcotic medication. I was desperate to find a safer alternative. I struggled with health-care providers over recommendations for operations, pain medication, and physical therapy. We all struggled with the issue of "What do we do next?"

> Chronic pain can be successfully treated by creatively combining existing chemical dependency and chronic pain treatment methods.

One purpose in writing this book is to share the answer to that question. My goal is to demonstrate that it is possible to have successful treatment by creatively combining existing chemical dependency and chronic pain treatment methods using the CENAPS® Model of Relapse Prevention Counseling and Denial Management Counseling as its foundation. APM did not fully develop overnight and, in fact, work on it continues to this day.

The maturing process began with the pioneering work of Dr. Jerry Callaway and Dr. Philip Mac. These two addiction medicine specialists had a vision that was ahead of its time. They were sure that someone with a chronic pain disorder who developed an addictive disorder needed to be treated for both conditions at the same time.

Because of my own chronic pain condition and my interest in helping this population, they asked me to be the primary therapist for their addiction pain treatment program. I was now working with patients who had lost almost all hope of ever having a normal life. Some of these people came into our program in wheelchairs or using crutches and canes as well as being addicted to their medication. As the result of the program many of them walked out under their own power, in a relatively short period of time, with the ability to manage their pain in a new and healthier manner. I began to develop my own vision of addiction-free pain treatment, and the APM system started to grow.

APM Stage Two:
Working with Chronic Pain Patients

APM continued to mature because of a team approach that included all disciplines. The basic approach was pragmatic: we looked for methods that worked. I developed and promoted special treatment plans for patients, some of which were quite unheard of in a chemical dependency treatment program.

On-site chiropractic visits were arranged. Two to three massage therapy sessions per week became an integral part of my patients' treatment plan. One of the more memorable activities included trips to a hydrotherapy treatment facility. In such a relaxed and nurturing environment patients were much more open and willing to share. In addition, I learned that exercising in water was much more beneficial than land-based workouts for many chronic pain conditions.

The APM System continued to grow with many challenges ahead.

Within the first few years I worked in the pain program, I noticed that many patients who were not in the pain program—and even some of the treatment staff—began to complain about the "special" treatment pain patients were receiving. Other staff thought the pain patients were complaining and "drug-seeking." At a time when teamwork was most needed, the staff was in constant conflict. I began to ask myself, "Now what?"

Fortunately, Drs. Callaway and Mac advocated for the pain program and helped me develop a plan to address these issues and facilitate a team approach. It wasn't easy. At times the specialized alternative treatments were not allowed—too disruptive to the treatment milieu was the rationale. Finally, we educated the staff and helped them to understand that the pain patients were not being treated "special," but that they had special needs that had to be addressed if they were to succeed in treatment.

A major problem for APM was the onset of managed care.

Another major problem for APM was the onset of insurance reform and the initial introduction of a managed care approach. This started in the name of cost containment, but resulted in many patients no longer receiving adequate treatment. When chemically dependent chronic pain patients do not receive effective treatment, they continue to overutilize the health-care system and their problems get even worse. Instead of containing costs, expenses grow even higher and some people can die as a result of not receiving adequate treatment. Even people who had started in our pain program experienced problems, despite the fact they were receiving effective treatment.

What made this process even more difficult was that a high percentage of the pain patients were dropping out of treatment at a much higher rate than other patients. It was at this time that I was first exposed to the Gorski-CENAPS® tools that one of the hospital's counselors, Molly Burke, brought back from her CENAPS® relapse prevention training. The one tool that made a huge difference in discouraging patients from leaving against medical advice was the **Relapse Prevention Early Intervention Plan.**

We interviewed patients and asked them to answer three questions:

- What are you going to do if you want to leave treatment?
- What should we as treatment providers do if you ask to leave treatment?
- Who are the significant people in your life who we can involve to help you get through the moments of craving and despair without leaving treatment?

Out of these questions we developed a concrete, specific plan of action that could be used to proactively intervene should patients want to leave treatment against medical advice. This plan allowed early identification and effective responses rather than patient management by crisis.

The more I learned about the Gorski-CENAPS® Model, the more intrigued I became. I realized this could be the way to increase the effectiveness of the pain program. As you will see in the following chapters, it turned out I was right.

Another problem associated with the long-term success of this population developed after they left primary treatment and went into a continuing care program. Many of the patients did not last more than three or four weeks before dropping out. Some of them ended up experiencing painful relapses and returning to treatment even more hopeless than before.

We struggled to find answers to this new dilemma. As it turned out, the answer was simple—but not easy. The pain patients needed their own continuing care program. The objections were loud, but I was not about to give up, so I volunteered to facilitate the first continuing care group for pain patients, realizing that effective treatment requires long-term, ongoing work.

> Relapse Prevention Tools are a crucial part of APM development.

While facilitating the continuing care group I learned the importance of ongoing warning sign identification and management. I knew I needed to understand more about relapse prevention to make a difference with this population. I didn't know it at the time, but my search for more relapse prevention tools was a crucial transition for the APM system and myself.

APM Stage Three:
Applying the CENAPS® Model

The big turning point for the APM system was a trip to Chicago to train with Terence Gorski at his Relapse Prevention Certification School. I was very excited when I first got there, but when I discovered what the next seven days were going to look like, I almost went back home. This was to be the most intense experiential training in which I had ever participated.

We attended lectures, practiced clinical techniques in role-play simulations, and worked on treatment applications in small groups. We had four primary jobs: learn the clinical model, integrate it with our clinical style, develop a plan to integrate it into our clinical programs, and learn how to appropriately adapt it to the needs of individual patients. By completing this rigorous training program and the optional competency certification, I learned how to skillfully apply relapse prevention therapy to the treatment of patients with addictive disorders and chronic pain conditions.

In going through the rigorous case-study process, I discovered ways to use my new skills with pain patients. I also realized I had to make a dramatic change in my career if I were ever going to really help people with chronic pain. So I resigned from my job at the hospital and went back to college. It was then that I started researching and writing about addiction-free pain management.

> Addiction-Free Pain Management grew from
> personal experience and the integration of
> treatment methods for chemical dependency,
> relapse prevention, and chronic pain.

While attending classes I continued to offer consultation services for other treatment professionals and started training others to work with pain and addiction issues. I assisted one of the local chemical dependency treatment hospitals to develop their own pain management program.

By this time I was implementing even more CENAPS® tools, such as identifying and managing high-risk situations, warning sign identification, and warning sign management. I was also using other ideas I had discovered in my research of pain clinic treatment programs. I started recommending ecclectic pain management approaches: acupuncture, trigger point injections, hypnotherapy, etc. These *holistic* approaches are covered in a later chapter.

> Combining the CENAPS® tools and holistic pain
> management approaches helped form the
> foundation for the existing APM model.

Combining the CENAPS® tools and holistic pain management approaches was a big step for APM—one that would help form the foundation for the existing model. I knew I was on the right path now. People I worked with in my private practice were getting effective treatment and avoiding relapse in growing numbers. But I knew we had a long way to go. I could envision the APM program in my mind but wondered how I could encourage other people to use the model?

It was at this point that fate intervened. I was scheduled to be on the CENAPS® faculty for another advanced certification training school, and had just completed a journal article on my vision of an effective treatment approach for people with chronic pain and addictive disorders. I asked Terence Gorski to read my article and give me feedback, which proved to be the beginning of our joint effort in formulating a relapse prevention workbook for this population.

Together we collaborated to design a system that would provide effective treatment for people with chronic pain and addiction issues. The development of *Addiction-Free Pain Management: A Relapse Prevention Counseling Workbook* began in April 1997, and in 1999 our second book, the *APM Professional Guide*, was published. Again a team approach was crucial to the process. Many other treatment professionals were needed to help the APM system through the next stage of development.

APM Stage Four:
Field-Testing the System

In addition to writing the workbook and professional guide, I also created a training process based on my years of research and clinical practice with this population. I was finally able to offer it to the world for other people to use.

The more I write, the more I train others, the more I learn myself. The evolution of APM is an ongoing process that becomes richer every time I teach a class, write an article, or work with my patients. The process is indeed coming of age. I envision this book as another of the major milestones in the development of the APM system.

The development of the APM Professional Guide began in December 1997 soon after the final submission of the *Addiction-Free Pain Management Workbook* to Herald House/Independence Press. It was then that Terry Gorski and I discussed the next project in the development of Addiction-Free Pain Management. He suggested that I begin writing a book that would serve two purposes: (1) to define and explain Addiction-Free Pain Management and (2) to explain how to get the full benefit from using the *Addiction-Free Pain Management Workbook.*

The development of this *Recovery Guide* first started when the *Professional Guide* was published in 1999, while at the same time developing a brochure and training entitled *Managing Pain Medication in Recovery.*

APM Stage Five:
Spreading the Word

Due to my personal and professional experiences, I know that successful treatment for people with chemical dependency and chronic pain can be achieved. You are all now a part of this work in progress.

By creatively combining the chemical dependency and chronic pain treatment methods presented in this *Recovery Guide* and the *Addiction-Free Pain Management Workbook* you can help spread a message of hope to other people who want help managing their chronic pain as you are learning to do.

For most of you the Addiction-Free Pain Management process will include using the eight **core clinical processes**. Some of you will also need the **medication management components**, and still others will need one or more of the **holistic treatment processes**. Many of you need a combination of all three components.

APM Core Clinical Processes

Addiction-Free Pain Management (APM) has an eight-part core clinical protocol for treating people with chronic pain disorders who also have addictive disorders. I call each part of the APM protocol a *clinical process.* To make consistent implementation of the process easier, faster, and more effective, I developed the *Addiction-Free Pain Management Workbook* that provides exercises related to each core clinical process. What follows is a brief description of each of these eight processes. The remainder of this book is primarily devoted to exploring how you can use these clinical processes more effectively as well as implementing the other two core components—**medication management** and **holistic components**.

External awareness leads to internal cognitive/ affective restructuring.

As you go through the remainder of this book and are learning how the *Addiction-Free Pain Management Workbook* is best used, please remember one important point. The major purpose of each of the workbook exercises is not just to "fill out the forms"; the goal is to increase your understanding about your condition and show you what it takes to heal the damage in the biopsychosocial areas of your life.

Process 1: The Effects of Chronic Pain

Many of you don't have the words you need to accurately describe the symptoms that you're experiencing. The purpose of this clinical process is to teach you a new vocabulary for describing your pain and its related symptoms. You will review and analyze a list of chronic pain symptoms, identify the symptoms of chronic pain that you're experiencing, and evaluate the severity of each symptom.

Process 2: The Effects of Prescription and/or Other Drugs

Many of you are using a variety of different medications to treat chronic pain and the underlying medical disorders that are causing the pain. This clinical process will help you understand the various medications used to treat your pain disorder by identifying the medications that you're currently using, and exploring the desired outcomes of using the medication. You will also learn to evaluate the benefits and disadvantages of using each medication.

Process 3: Decision Making about Pain Medication

In this process you will explore the reasons why you started using problematic pain medication (including alcohol) and other drugs. You are then instructed to make an assessment of life damaging problems you experienced as a result of using chemicals, and explore the reasons for deciding to stop using them.

Process 4: Abstinence Contract and Intervention Planning

In this clinical process you are asked to make a commitment to abstinence and to develop a recovery plan. You will complete and sign an abstinence contract, agreeing to maintain abstinence from any *inappropriate* pain medication. You are then instructed to develop a relapse intervention plan that describes the responsibilities of yourself, your counselor, and at least two or three significant others to help stop relapse quickly should it occur.

Process 5: Identifying and Personalizing High-Risk Situations

In this clinical process you learn to identify the immediate high-risk situations that can cause chemical use and ineffective pain management in spite of your commitment. You are instructed to review a list of common high-risk situations that can activate the urge to use/abuse problematic pain medication (including alcohol) or other drugs and/or to sabotage your effective pain management program. You are then asked to identify and personalize your own most important (critical) high-risk situation and write a personal title and description for use in self-monitoring.

Process 6: Mapping High-Risk Situations

In this clinical process you are asked to describe one past situation in which you experienced your immediate high-risk situation in recovery and managed it poorly. This situation map will be used to help you identify the pattern of self-defeating behaviors that drive the relapse process. You are then instructed to identify one past situation in which you experienced your immediate high-risk situation in recovery and managed it effectively. This situation will be used to identify new and more effective ways of coping with your future high-risk situations. These new behaviors will become the foundation for High-Risk Situation Management and Recovery Planning.

Process 7: Analyzing and Managing High-Risk Situations

In this clinical process you are asked to analyze the immediate high-risk situation that you're learning to manage. You are asked to identify the irrational (addictive) **thoughts**, unmanageable **feelings**, self-destructive **urges**, self-defeating (addictive) **actions**, and **reactions** of others (TFUARs), that drive your high-risk situation. You are shown how to manage this kind of high-risk situation more appropriately by identifying three points where you can use more effective ways of thinking, feeling, and acting to avoid relapse. You are then instructed to apply these new ways of coping to a future high-risk situation.

Process 8: Recovery Planning

In this clinical process you are asked to develop a schedule of recovery activities that will support the ongoing identification and effective management of your high-risk situations. You are then instructed to write a schedule of recovery activities and explore how each activity can be adapted to help you identify and manage your high-risk situations.

APM Medication Management Components

Some pain disorders require pharmacological (prescription drug) interventions. Other conditions may respond to over-the-counter medications like aspirin and ibuprofen. Still other conditions need a combination of both.

However, some pain disorders can be treated without any pharmacological interventions. These other treatment approaches are called **Holistic Treatment Processes** and will be described at the end of this chapter.

I have included a chart (provided by Dr. Mark Stanford), followed by a narrative description of the pharmacological interventions. I will show the medications used, how they work, and for which conditions they are typically used.

MEDICATION USES	MECHANISM OF ACTION (HOW THEY WORK)	TREATMENT USES
1. NON-NARCOTIC ANALGESICS: ASPIRIN, ACETAMINOPHEN (TYLENOL), IBUPROFEN	Act mostly on the peripheral nervous system. Inhibits prostaglandin E, a substance that sensitizes pain receptors, and increases body pain receptors, inflammation, and body temperature.	Headaches, muscle pain analgesia, anti-inflammatory, anti-pyretic (fever reducer)
2. NARCOTIC ANALGESICS: CODEINE, MORPHINE, DEMEROL	Act in central nervous system to block pain messages. Activate pain modulating systems in the brain that project to the spinal cord. Block signals from descending nerve pathways that inhibit the neurons and thus reduce the intensity of pain sensation. Many types of narcotic analgesics.	Post-operative pain, other pain conditions
3. NARCOTIC AND NON-NARCOTIC COMBINATIONS OTHER PAIN-REDUCING DRUGS	Act on a variety of neurotransmitter systems. Sometimes a combination of narcotics with non-narcotic analgesics such as Percocet (percodan and acetaminophen) or Vicoprofen (vicodan and ibuprofen).	Variety of pain conditions
4. ANTIDEPRESSANT DRUGS (I.E. TRICYCLICS)	Increase activity of certain neurotransmitters.	Chronic pain, atypical pain syndromes
5. EPIDURAL INJECTIONS	Reduction of inflammation in the spine (usually surrounding a damaged spinal disc producing pain). Certain steroid drugs (drugs related to cortisone) that contain strong anti-inflammatory properties.	Inflammatory pain from damaged spinal disc, arthritic spinal joints, acute strain of spinal muscles or ligaments, pain caused by degeneration of the spine as in osteoporosis

1. Non-Narcotic Analgesics

The non-narcotic analgesics include medications such as aspirin, acetaminophen (Tylenol), and ibuprofen (Motrin, Advil). These medications relieve pain by acting on your peripheral nervous system.

The non-narcotic analgesics inhibit the production of a chemical substance called prostaglandin E. Prostaglandin E is released in response to an initial pain stimulus. Prostaglandin E intensifies your pain in four ways.

- First, it makes your body's pain receptors more sensitive.
- Second, it increases the number of your body's pain receptors.
- Third, it causes inflammation, which in turn creates a new source for your pain.
- Fourth, it elevates your body temperature creating the pain and discomfort that comes along with having a fever.

Because non-narcotic analgesics inhibit the production of prostaglandin E they reduce these pain-inducing reactions. As a result the non-narcotic analgesics are a medication of choice for the treatment of headaches, muscle pain, inflammation, and fever.

2. Narcotic Analgesics

The narcotic analgesics act within your central nervous system to block pain messages. Narcotics activate pain-modulating systems that are projected from your brain to your spinal cord, which block signals from descending nerve pathways that inhibit specific neurons, thereby reducing the intensity of your pain sensation. There are many types of narcotic analgesics. The best known include codeine, morphine, and Demerol (meperidine).

The narcotic analgesics are used for the treatment of intense pain. They are ideal for treating postoperative pain and severe pain conditions caused by acute injury. Most people develop tolerance to the pain-killing affects within eight to twelve weeks and require an increase in dosage. As a result, narcotics are highly addictive. They should be used with extreme caution and are not usually the medication of choice for the treatment of mild to moderate, long-term (chronic) pain conditions.

3. Narcotic and Non-Narcotic Combinations

There are a variety of other pain-reducing drugs. Many of these are a combination of narcotic with non-narcotic analgesics. These combinations can provide the pain-relieving benefits of both types of painkillers and act on a variety of neurotransmitter systems. Some of the common combinations of narcotics and non-narcotic analgesics include Percocet (a combination of percodan and acetaminophen), Vicoprofen (a combination hydrocodone and ibuprofen), and Tylenol 3 (a combination of Tylenol with Codeine).

Because of the wide variety of pain-relieving effects, the narcotic and non-narcotic combinations are used in a wide variety of pain conditions that exhibit a combination of Type 1 (direct) and Type 2 (indirect) pain characteristics.

4. Antidepressant Drugs

Antidepressant drugs may be indicated for several reasons. One reason is that many people with chronic pain disorders become clinically depressed. Once again the APM approach indicates that an evaluation by a specialist is needed to determine the severity of the problem.

Some types of depression (situational) respond best to cognitive behavioral therapy. Other types (bipolar) may need a pharmacological intervention. There are many different types or classifications of antidepressants to choose from, so a specialist should be consulted to determine the most effective choice for you.

There is another important factor for considering using an antidepressant: pain reduction. The use of tricyclic antidepressants has been an effective tool in pain management for years. For example the tricyclic amitriptyline is frequently used to treat and help prevent migraine headaches. These antidepressants have been able to provide relief for nerve pain and often result in lowering the dose of narcotic medications.

5. Epidural Injections

Epidural injection is the process of administering a drug into the outer covering of your central nervous system, usually in the spine. The use of epidural steroid injections can lead to a reduction of inflammation in your spine (usually surrounding a damaged spinal disc). Certain steroid drugs (drugs related to cortisone) contain strong anti-inflammatory properties. This reduction in inflammation leads to a decrease in pain.

The use of opioids injected epidurally can lead to significant pain relief for severe pain conditions. This technique uses a lower dose of opioid, which has a longer duration and no risk of sedation. However, sometimes side effects may occur, so this procedure is usually reserved for serious conditions in a specialized care center.

APM Holistic Treatment Components

Non-pharmacological treatments have also been shown to be effective for some pain conditions. Recent studies have shown that endorphins mediate the analgesic effects of acupuncture and placebos as well. Still to be discovered is the mechanism by which hypnosis accomplishes its analgesic effects.

Addiction-Free Pain Management uses both the core clinical components and the medication management components described earlier as well as the holistic processes described below. Because each of you has your own unique problems and needs that may not be covered here, be assured that there are more than just the seven holistic approaches listed below that are available for you. The remainder of this book describes how to effectively implement both the core and optional components to obtain the best outcome for you.

1. Meditation and Relaxation

For decades the chemical dependency literature has demonstrated the effectiveness of teaching meditation and relaxation techniques to people with addictive disorders. The pain literature also indicates the importance of using relaxation to help reduce the level of pain people experience.

There are many books and audiocassettes that can teach you how to use meditation and relaxation exercises to reduce stress and anxiety. Later I will discuss the stress-pain connection. Meanwhile remember that in most cases if you can learn to lower your stress levels, you will also experience a decrease in your level of pain.

2. Emotional Management

Most chemical dependency treatment professionals realize the importance of teaching their patients how to appropriately deal with emotional issues to reduce their stress and anxiety. The CENAPS® model is based in part on the belief that avoiding painful emotions will often lead a recovering chemically dependent person to relapse.

One of the most difficult, and most crucial, emotional issues that must be resolved is your grief and loss of health and/or prior level of functioning. You can accomplish this essential task by working with a qualified counselor or therapist.

3. Massage Therapy and Physical Therapy

As I mentioned earlier, direct pressure could sometimes change the way you experience pain. When using massage therapy it's important to realize that there will be some immediate pain relief and reduced muscle tension, but it will be short-lived if not followed with other measures. This is understandable because there are many precursors or triggers for muscle tension that often resurface soon after the massage session. Therefore, other measures must be implemented that are specific to your needs and used in the proper sequence.

Many health-care providers promote the combination of physical therapy and hydrotherapy in addition to the massage therapy to help you learn how to strengthen and recondition your body, thus you become an active participant in your healing process.

4. Chiropractic Treatment

Many people with chronic pain receive long-term pain reduction when undergoing chiropractic treatment. Chiropractic adjustments restore proper motion and function to your damaged joints, thereby reducing irritation to associated muscles and nerves.

Most chiropractors are trained in nutrition and many include dietary changes and nutrient supplementation in their treatment plans. This process helps to build up the immune system while at the same time raising your pain threshold. A later chapter discusses the importance of using supplements as part of your healing process.

5. Acupuncture

Acupuncture is often effective in managing certain types of pain for three reasons. First, acupuncture stimulates the large nerve fibers that inhibit pain signalling. Second, acupuncture may produce a placebo effect through the release of endorphins and enkephalins. Third, acupuncture may stimulate small nerve fibers and inhibit spinal cord pain signaling. Acupuncture is often used in the treatment of back pain, minor surgery, and other pain conditions.

6. Biofeedback

Biofeedback has proven to be another effective "active" method that you can learn so that you can participate further in your own treatment. This procedure teaches you how to let go of your stress and tension.

Effective biofeedback treatment is progressive and includes several steps. The treatment starts with an accurate diagnosis of your problem followed by implementation of the proper treatment modality. It also includes time for you to practice situations that simulate instances in which the symptoms most often arise. Learning to use meditation and relaxation techniques to reduce stress is also a helpful complement to the biofeedback process.

7. Hypnosis

Hypnosis can be an effective treatment for various pain conditions. There is some evidence that certain people are more susceptible to the effects of hypnosis than others. The effects of hypnosis are definitely biopsychosocial. Although we're not certain how hypnosis biologically mediates pain, there is growing evidence that hypnosis may activate pain-inhibitory descending nerve pathways from your brain to your spinal cord. It appears, however, that hypnosis does not affect the opioid pathways.

Hypnosis also creates an altered state of consciousness that is usually marked by a slowing of brain wave patterns. As a result people under the influence of hypnosis often experience a state of consciousness associated with alpha and theta brain wave activity. These states of consciousness bypass normal cognitive processes and hence can prevent many expectancies and beliefs about the pain experience from coming to your mind. This is a useful intervention for *anticipatory pain,* which I covered earlier.

Psychologically, hypnosis may act in your brain to shift attention away from pain sensations. Hypnosis is commonly used in conjunction with dental procedures, childbirth, burns, and headaches.

Socially, hypnosis may create a cultural expectation through suggestion that the pain will be minimal and manageable. The social context of hypnotic suggestion may also distract from the pain.

APM works in the real world with real people.

Now the challenge is to understand how to adapt the information in this chapter to work for you in the real world. The remainder of this book will take you through the APM process with two of my patients, Donna and Matt (names and other identifying information have been changed to protect their confidentiality).

Chapter Four

Learning to Live Again

Understanding Your Chronic Pain

Chronic pain can be difficult to treat. Your pain is real. Your need for relief is urgent. The typical treatment involves the use of narcotics so you may be at a high risk of becoming addicted to your pain medications. When undergoing pain management treatment you may need to ask yourself a series of difficult questions.

- What if the traditional medication management doesn't work?
- What if I quickly develop tolerance to my pain medication and require progressively larger doses to gain pain relief?
- What will I do if I consistently abuse my pain medication either by increasing the dosage or taking it more often than prescribed?
- How will I distinguish whether I legitimately need more pain medication over a longer period of time or have become addicted to my medication?
- How will I deal with my feelings of helplessness and hopelessness because I'm in pain and/or have become addicted to my pain medications and can see no way out?

The Addiction-Free Pain Management (APM) system provides a way to answer these and many other difficult questions that are routinely asked by people with chronic pain. As I mentioned previously, the APM system is a treatment approach that uses the Gorski-CENAPS® biopsychosocial model.

The APM System integrates the most advanced pain management methods developed at the nation's leading pain clinics, with the most effective treatment methods for addiction developed at the nation's leading chemical dependency treatment programs. The result is a unique integration of treatment methods that combine proper medication management with non-pharmacological techniques. This leads to pain relief, while lowering or eliminating your risk of addiction or relapse.

How Donna & Matt Deal with Their Pain

I am using two former patients, Donna and Matt, to illustrate the various APM methods that I describe. The remainder of this book is designed to help you to accomplish the following:

- understand the APM treatment methods;
- integrate APM methods into your personal recovery program; and
- adapt APM methods to meet the unique needs of your personal life.

Each concept of the APM system is explained and then I describe how these methods were applied with two very different patients. By doing this you can see the different levels at which you can apply the APM methods to yourself.

The following chapters explore the separate elements of APM by showing how Donna and Matt completed the APM process and by discussing the exercises in the *Addiction-Free Pain Management Workbook*. Donna and Matt are typical of the many people who experience the combination of chemical dependency and chronic pain. Now, I would like to introduce you to Donna and Matt.

Introducing Donna

People in chronic pain often seek treatment as a result of a complex combination of physical, psychological, and social problems. Serious issues can complicate effective treatment and need to be addressed in order to successfully manage a pain disorder. Donna's case is no exception.

Donna is a thirty-five-year-old married woman, mother of a teenage son by a previous marriage and two daughters under age five with her current husband. Donna's teenage son is actively chemically dependent and her spouse is physically, verbally, and emotionally abusive. As a result, she is living in conditions that are stressful and interfere with her ability to manage her chronic pain. This increases the likelihood of her abusing medication in order to get emotional relief from the difficult circumstances of her environment.

Donna has suffered from ongoing abdominal pain since she was a young teenager. The pain started after a much older male relative physically and sexually abused her. She has current flashbacks to those abusive incidents,

Donna is obsessive-compulsive and has a tendency to act out by using repetitive behaviors that have little or nothing to do with helping her to solve the immediate problems she is facing. As a result, a central focus of her treatment has been to help her to pause when facing a problem and select a relevant response that can help her to solve the problem, rather than act out repetitive, self-defeating behaviors.

Donna's father has a prescription drug dependency, and he often encouraged her to take addictive medications. Donna has an extremely difficult time with trust and is very resistant to self-help groups. This is compounded by the fact that her first husband was also abusive to her and to her son.

> It is cruicial to build on the initial motivation for treatment.

Donna's motivation for treatment came from a referral by her primary care physician, who insisted that she be in pain management therapy if he was to continue prescribing pain medication for her abdominal pain.

Introducing Matt

Matt is a fifty-year-old divorced male who has a long history of addictive disorders. He has been in more than twenty addiction treatment programs during the past fifteen years. Matt has several physical problems; most critical is a serious back injury as a result of a construction accident more than ten years ago.

He finally admitted to his doctor and to himself that he was really taking pain medication to help him to cope with uncomfortable feelings and to get high (experience that pleasant state of euphoria), which would help him to forget about his problems for a little while. Matt also experienced extreme shame about past sexual trauma that causes sexual dysfunction, which he believes led to his divorce and currently blocks him from entering a healthy intimate relationship.

> Isolation tendencies are common with chronic pain and addictive disorders.

Matt has a tendency to isolate when in legitimate pain (either physical or emotional) and often found himself at urgent care clinics where it was easy for him to persuade the staff to give him narcotic medication for his multiple physical pain symptoms.

Matt's motivation for treatment was the result of his primary care physician refusing to treat him after his latest relapse unless he underwent relapse prevention therapy.

Learning to Connect

Both Donna and Matt share the same lack of trust found in many chemically dependent chronic pain patients. Many of you may have been given negative messages from your caregivers. Messages like "It's all in your head," "You need to try harder," "It can't be that bad," or maybe "You're making yourself hurt so you can get drugs," or the infamous "You'll just have to learn to live with it."

Due to these negative messages, combined with feelings of hopelessness and helplessness, you may have become very guarded and defensive. Finding an effective way to connect is a crucial part of APM treatment success. In the intervention planning and recovery planning sections you will learn how to incorporate other people into your APM team.

The Initial Decision

Your initial decision to seek help is the most crucial point in your treatment process. Finding treatment providers who are willing to work with you, not on you, is also important. It's helpful to find doctors, therapists, or counselors who are willing to understand you as a whole person, not just a pain condition.

Make an Empowered Decision

Answering the following five questions as completely and honestly as possible can help you to make or reinforce your decision to start the APM process:

1. What is the *best* that will happen if I continue using my pain medication and managing my pain the way I have been doing?
2. What is the *worst* that will happen if I continue using my pain medication and managing my pain the way I have been doing?
3. What is the *worst* that will happen if I decide to start on this APM recovery journey?
4. What is the *best* that will happen if I decide to start on this APM recovery journey?
5. What am I *willing* to do to complete this APM process and develop a plan to overcome any resistance or obstacles?

Once you answer these five questions you will have the information you need to make an empowered decision and develop an action plan to move forward. It's imperative that you not try to do this work alone for many reasons. The most important reason is that many times people in chronic pain, or those who develop substance abuse/dependency, tend to isolate themselves. Another good reason is that **you deserve to have support** when dealing with this problem. The APM process requires a tremendous amount of hard work and self-honesty, as well as including other people on your *team* who are willing—and able—to support you in a healthy way.

It's important to note that if you are currently using your pain medication problematically or experiencing negative consequences from the medication, you may need detoxification treatment before starting the APM treatment process. Some of you may not have reached the abuse or dependency stages yet, but you can also benefit from the APM process so you do not have to experience the full weight of addiction.

Detoxification Issues

Neurotransmitters and Pain Suppression

When people become addicted to their pain medication, their brains develop a tolerance so that their medication no longer works as it was originally intended. This is the reason detoxification is necessary. To understand how this happens we need to look at how neurotransmitters and pain suppression function. Stimulation of certain areas of the brain can cause pain suppression. In the brain, there are a variety of chemicals called neurotransmitters—substances that transmit information to the brain and body. Three neurotransmitters—enkephalins, serotonin, and endorphins—are known to be associated with pain suppression.

Analgesic treatments (treatments that prevent pain) are believed to be assisted by endorphins and enkephalins. Consistent with this understanding, it is currently believed that opiates relieve pain because they are similar in structure to endorphins and enkephalins, and therefore act on the same sites in your brain and spinal cord as do these neurotransmitters.

> Increased use of opiates leads to a decrease in your natural endorphins and enkephalins.

Because opiates are so similar in their chemical structure to neurotransmitters, there is a concern that using them repeatedly over a period of time will reduce the quantity of your brain's natural pain suppressant neurotransmitters. With repeated use of opiates, your brain responds and adapts by slowing down production of its own natural opiates (the endorphins/enkephalins), which are more effective for pain suppression than synthetic narcotics. In a sense, the brain begins to adapt to the presence of an opiate drug by reducing its own natural source of pain suppressing neurotransmitters. The result is that opiate drugs can ultimately increase the sensation of pain via the brain's adaptive response—this is sometimes called a pain-rebound effect.

Neurotransmitters and Withdrawal

When someone who abuses narcotic analgesics abruptly stops taking these drugs, they often experience a hypersensitive, painful physical reaction. This is why the narcotic withdrawal syndrome can be so uncomfortable and painful. It takes approximately two weeks for the brain to "de-adapt" from using opiate medication—which has essentially replaced its own pain-reducing capacity—and go back to its own ability to make and use endorphins.

Because of the potential for physical dependency (meaning that the drug produces tolerance and a characteristic withdrawal syndrome upon abrupt cessation of use), opiate medications should only be used with the highest degree of caution in persons experiencing chronic pain disorders.

How and where to start treatment varies depending on the results of the identification and assessment process I discussed earlier. However, effective treatment cannot be obtained if you remain on problematic pain medication (including alcohol). In APM treatment the first approach is often detoxification and stabilization.

Inpatient vs. Outpatient

Sometimes this stage of treatment needs to incorporate an inpatient program due to the quantity and/or types of medication being used. In other situations, an outpatient detoxification protocol can be effectively implemented. Whatever method is used, it should be implemented with the team approach in mind. You need to be an integral part of this team because empowering yourself is essential in order to obtain a positive treatment outcome.

A major early treatment difference between pain clinics and CD (chemical dependency) treatment centers involves medication and detoxification issues. Although many pain clinics do withdraw their patients from most narcotic medication, some do not. Meanwhile, most CD treatment professionals believe that chemical dependency is a chronic, life-threatening disease. Therefore, they conclude that the removal of all psychoactive chemicals is imperative for effective treatment. If the progression of the addictive disorder is not too advanced, an outpatient detoxification protocol could be used.

Even when there is agreement on detoxification as the starting point for recovery treatment, how that task is accomplished may vary. For many medications it can be dangerous to have the person suddenly quit taking the medication without medical precautions. Often those precautions include other medication to ensure a safe withdrawal. Below are two examples of detoxification. If you need to be medically detoxified, make sure you learn as much about the process as possible—this is called informed consent.

Two Approaches for Detoxification

In chemical dependency (CD) treatment centers there are basically two methods typically used for administering detoxification medication: (a) on an as-needed (or PRN) basis, and (b) a regular interval administration. One drawback of the PRN method is that you can still self-medicate, while a drawback of option b is that it may result in your experiencing high levels of pain before each dose is due. Although physician prescription of analgesics in sufficient doses may be preferable, a compromise solution would consist of an as-needed order with a range of doses, depending on your level of pain.

In many pain clinics the **pain cocktail method** is used for withdrawing people from the problem drug(s). This technique allows the gradual and systematic withdrawal of analgesics, narcotics, or benzodiazepines.

The process involves combining the detoxification medication into a single mix, which is given in a disguising mixture (such as cherry syrup). The mix is given only at fixed time intervals on an ongoing basis. The decrease in medication is achieved by gradually withdrawing the active ingredients, while keeping the total volume the same.

> You need to be proactive in your own healing process.

However, one difficulty with the pain cocktail approach is that it keeps you in a passive role. The APM approach encourages you to take a proactive part in your treatment, which includes being informed about the exact parameters of your detoxification protocol.

Detoxification for Donna and Matt

Now let's look at the approaches used when Donna and Matt went through their detoxification.

> ## Matt needed inpatient detoxification.

Matt's last relapse started when he abused a nonsteroidal anti-inflammatory medication, Ultram (tramadol). This medication is contraindicated for patients with a history of opiate dependency or abuse, and in Matt's case it re-triggered his addiction. In fact, he was using more than ten times the recommended dose when he finally sought help.

Part of this re-triggering effect occurred when Matt sought help at urgent care clinics to obtain Vicodin, which he also started abusing. In addition, he was using a benzodiazapine medication for his anxiety. This relapse episode was the first time Matt admitted to using medication for emotional pain as well as for physical pain symptoms.

Matt's early treatment plan included not only detoxification and stabilization, but also training in emotional management skills. With Matt's combination and quantity of drug use, an addiction medicine practitioner determined that inpatient treatment was the safest modality.

> ## Donna's case was much different. She needed an outpatient protocol.

Donna's motivation for treatment was an external intervention. Her primary care physician insisted that she be in pain management psychotherapy if he were to continue prescribing pain medication for her abdominal pain (gastroenteritis).

Because she was on more of a maintenance level of medication, her physician was open to outpatient medication management with the long-term goal being the eventual elimination of all narcotic pain medication.

This was frightening for Donna, who did not believe she could ever function without her pain medication. Because a very toxic and stressful living environment amplified Donna's pain symptoms, one early approach included teaching Donna how to manage her stress more effectively.

Finding safer medication is crucial.

The ongoing use of pain medication may be a necessary treatment alternative for some people. However, narcotic medication is usually contraindicated for most chronic pain conditions due to the tendency of the user to develop tolerance. When you do need to be on narcotic medications you must have an effective plan in place. Earlier I discussed the importance of understanding the pharmacological implications in determining the proper medication for ongoing chronic pain conditions. Once again, it's imperative that a team approach be used.

The importance of finding the safest medication possible cannot be overemphasized when narcotic medication is taken in increasingly larger doses due to tolerance, as the side affects from the medication may become life-threatening. It can be a long and arduous journey and is best accomplished with a guide and other companions.

Support Systems

Building Trust and Safety

Another potential block to effective treatment for Donna was her difficulty in trusting others and her resistance to using self-help groups. Finding the correct type of a support system was difficult for her, but she finally chose a support group for women near her home. Once she got to know the other women in the group, she reported feeling like she finally had a family that she might be able to trust.

Building trust and safety is a key part of any therapeutic process, but with the APM population it is even more important. Many of you have learned that it's not safe to trust healthcare providers and that many providers were not really listening to your complaints or taking your condition seriously.

On the other hand, many people who experience chronic pain conditions despise well-meaning, sympathetic people who may come across as patronizing. Such treatment tends to keep you in a victim role. Donna was especially hypervigilant in this regard. Matt had his own issues with trust and safety and had a tendency to isolate when life became difficult.

Using Twelve-Step Support

While Matt was willing, and even eager, to use Twelve-Step support groups, Donna was very reluctant. She believed she did not fit in at those meetings and chose a Christian recovering support group for women instead, although at first she was unable to open up until she developed trust in the group and felt safe to share.

In contrast, Matt tended to avoid his Twelve-Step support groups when he needed them the most. This resistance to seeking social support was an important obstacle for both of them to overcome.

Matt and Donna are not unique among chemically dependent, chronic pain patients who tend to avoid Twelve-Step support groups. Many of you may not believe that you are real addicts, and therefore think that you don't belong in those kinds of groups. That is why getting a professional assessment is so crucial.

Well-Intentioned but Dangerous Messages

As I discussed in chapter one, another obstacle you may experience, especially for those of you who must remain on some type of medication, are the confusing and conflicting messages at AA (Alcoholics Anonymous) or NA (Narcotic Anonymous) meetings.

The message you may hear says that in order to "belong," you must stop using everything—no matter what. This is not the official position of either of these programs. However, well-meaning, recovering alcoholics and addicts have sabotaged many a person's recovery process with these all-or-nothing messages as we saw earlier with Dave's story.

Precautions when Using Twelve-Step Support

I have seen a number of people with chronic pain and addictive disorders receive inappropriate advice from their recovery programs. These situations are frustrating because they are so unnecessary and can easily lead to relapse and in some cases even death.

You need to be aware that this could happen to you. You need to be prepared to deal with well-meaning people. It would be helpful to seek out the Alcoholics Anonymous conference-approved pamphlet that clearly explains that some members need to be on *appropriate* medication.

Taking medication is a serious concern for someone in recovery, but as I explained earlier, sometimes medication is necessary for certain chronic pain conditions. This is where the medication management components of APM are useful.

Using Pills Anonymous and Pain Support Groups

There is another Twelve-Step program that may be more appropriate for addicted chronic pain people who have developed problems due to pain medication use. This program is called Pills Anonymous (PA).

Other communities may have chronic pain support groups that are also beneficial for APM patients. Group therapy and peer support groups have proven to be effective components for successful treatment outcomes and should be sought out.

Support groups and therapy groups also provide another essential component—non-pharmacological pain management education and stress reduction tools. Both Donna and Matt were finally able to connect and stay with appropriate peer support groups.

Getting Started: Transition and Stabilization Tasks

Once you are actually in treatment and have gone through detoxification or are being withdrawn from the problem medication, you are in what the CENAPS® Developmental Model of Recovery refers to as the Transition and Stabilization Stages of Recovery that I mentioned earlier.

According to the CENAPS® model there are five important tasks that you need to accomplish during these stages:

- Recovering physically from the withdrawal effects of chemicals
- Working through resistance and denial
- Discontinuing preoccupation with chemicals
- Learning to solve problems without using chemicals
- Developing hope and motivation for recovery

To give you the best hope of rapidly accomplishing these transitional tasks, you need to quickly integrate yourself into a recovery milieu. This is another point where identifying and managing your denial is important.

> Trust and safety are crucial.

As I discussed earlier, building trust and safety is important to help you fit in and bond. Many of you have learned to distrust others as a result of your dysfunctional family systems or other life events. You may have become isolated by the time you are ready to enter treatment. Some of you may even exhibit paranoid and/or agoraphobic (fear of going out) symptoms.

Letting go of your denial and other defenses through education and information, while at the same time learning to trust others, enables you to become capable of admitting and accepting your substance abuse or dependency. You can then identify with others in the treatment program or support groups, which helps you transition smoothly into recovery.

For some of you this process can be accomplished using group therapy followed by individual sessions on an as-needed basis. There is help available and a system that can lead you out of the problem and into the solution. This solution is described in the following chapters, showing you how the APM system works.

Now that you have an extensive overview of addiction, the addiction-pain syndrome, and pain, you can begin the APM process. What follows next is an overview of the APM process and how to get the most out of the APM workbook. At this point it would be very helpful for you to begin working in the APM workbook as you go through the remainder of the recovery guide.

Chapter Five

Beginning the APM Process

The Effects of Chronic Pain

When recovering from a pain disorder it's essential to understand the difference between acute pain and chronic pain, especially when you may need to manage your pain with potentially addictive medication. As I mentioned in chapter two, it is also very important for you to understand the biopsychosocial impact your chronic pain condition has on you.

In the following section I describe the three parts of Process One in the APM workbook that are designed to assist you to identify the biopsychosocial properties of your pain.

Process One, Part 1: Acute Pain vs. Chronic Pain

This process explains the difference between acute pain and chronic pain as well as describing the biopsychosocial effects of pain. The primary goal of this exercise is to increase your knowledge and understanding of pain and its effects to help you move from victimization to empowerment.

As I mentioned earlier, pain can be classified as either acute or chronic. Because the conditions are so different, the treatment of acute pain is different from the treatment of chronic pain. It's important to know the difference and to be able to learn how to have a specific management plan for each.

Acute Pain

Earlier I described how acute pain tells you that something has gone wrong or that damage to the system has occurred. The source of the pain can usually be easily identified, and typically acute pain does not last very long. Acute pain is a symptom of an immediate underlying problem.

An example of acute pain is when you touch a hot burner on the stove. Your first reaction is to pull away your hand. Contact with the heat will leave you with symptoms from minor redness to serious tissue damage, but in each acute pain case there is a predictable period of time for the burn to heal. There are also effective medical treatments that promote quick healing. Some other causes of acute pain include cuts and bro-

---

Acute Pain

- An immediate signal to the brain
- Signals damage dysfunction
- Is readily treatable
- Is of limited duration

---

ken bones.

No matter what the source of acute pain, the result is to drive you to search for relief. Once the problem is identified, it's customary—and usually safe unless you have a history of substance abuse or dependency—to use analgesic and/or narcotic medication for acute pain relief. If you are in recovery for chemical dependency, you should consult an addiction medicine practitioner/specialist before any narcotic or psychoactive prescriptions are taken. You should also use an effective medication management plan, which I describe in chapter nine.

Chronic Pain

Chronic pain is a condition that fails to respond to standard medical interventions. In some cases there is no easily recognized reason for the pain, or the original acute condition seems to be resolved but the pain signals keep firing. In addition, the pain has a duration of three to six months. In many cases chronic pain no longer serves a useful purpose.

Matt and Donna present fairly typical examples of chronic pain conditions. Matt has chronic back pain. Although surgery and physical therapy have effectively treated the original injury, Matt's pain symptoms continued for years after his accident. Like many people with chronic pain, Matt was often told the pain was in his head. But to Matt the pain was very real—

Chronic Pain

- Fails to respond to typical treatments
- Sometimes has no recognized source
- Duration of at least three to six months
- May no longer serve a useful purpose

---

and he wanted relief!

Some other common chronic pain conditions include phantom limb pain, headaches, neck pain, and fibromyalgia. In chapter two I presented a more in-depth explanation of pain that was designed to help you get the most out of this part of the APM treatment process.

Biopsychosocial Effects of Chronic Pain

While you can generally receive effective medical care for acute pain, treatment for chronic pain can be a confusing process of misunderstanding and incorrect diagnoses.

When you experience chronic pain and doctors are at a loss to define the exact nature of your problem, you might start to believe you're going crazy. Often treatment professionals will validate that belief because they can find no observable reason for the symptoms. However, chronic pain is real and often occurs for reasons that may not be identified easily. As I explained earlier, chronic pain affects you physically, psychologically, and socially.

- Physically, chronic pain raises your stress level and drains physical energy.
- Psychologically, chronic pain affects your ability to think clearly, logically, and rationally, as well as to effectively manage feelings and emotions.
- Socially, chronic pain affects your ability to use consistently responsible behaviors, thus affecting your pain man-

Chronic Pain Affects Your	
Body	Thoughts
Emotions	Behaviors
Relationships	Pain Management

agement and other people.

In addition, the way that you sense or experience pain—its intensity and duration—will affect how well you are able to manage it. This goes back to our original discussion on pain versus suffering. Pain is an unpleasant signal telling you that something is wrong with your body. Suffering results from the meaning or interpretation you assign to the pain. Learning more positive ways of thinking about your pain will lead to more effective pain management.

When you have chronic pain it's usually accepted that something is physically wrong with your body. The symptoms of pain can range from mildly irritating, to somewhat annoying or uncomfortable, to moderately distressing, to severely horrible, to the worst possible excruciating suffering!

While you are affected biologically, other parts of you are also impacted. Your thought processes are affected in several different ways. Sometimes you might have difficulty thinking clearly or concentrating, which leads to an inability to solve problems that are normally easy for you. At times you may be unable to function very well in virtually all areas of your life. Instead of thinking positively you may repress certain thoughts and blank out, or indulge in self-defeating, negative thinking.

Chronic pain can also lead to difficulty in managing emotions. Sometimes you may be cut off from your emotions, become numb and not know what you are feeling. At other times you may overreact to your emotions. The intensity of your feel-

Chronic pain often leads to depression.

ings does not match the trigger situation.

In addition, many people with chronic pain frequently become depressed. When your thinking is irrational or dysfunctional and you are mismanaging your feelings, you can have urges to indulge in self-defeating impulsive or compulsive behaviors to cope with your distress. This, in turn, affects your relationships with others. Some of you may become isolated and believe you can handle life without any help, or you may become increasingly dependent on others to take care of you. This caretaking by others may be enabling you to continue self-defeating behaviors and keep you in a victim role.

The Biopsychosocial Sensation of Chronic Pain

Most people with chronic pain do not have the words they need to describe their pain. The first step in healing is to learn the words—a pain vocabulary—that you can learn to use to let others know about the type of pain you are experiencing. Remember that pain is a biopsychosocial experience. As a result you need to learn to make a distinction between the physical sensation of pain, your psychological interpretation of the pain, and how you use your pain in relationships with other people.

Process One, Part 2: Biopsychosocial Sensation of Chronic Pain

Over the past two decades I have reviewed several different pain assessment instruments (such as the McGuill Pain Assessment Questionnaire). I have used these instruments with patients, and through an active listening process I identified the sixty words that most of my patients found useful in describing their pain. I call these words the **pain vocabulary**.

In order to help you quickly find the words that describe your pain, the words are organized into twenty categories with three words in each category that progress from less severe to more severe pain.

When you have chronic pain your sensation of pain and its effects vary. Process One, Part 2: The Biopsychosocial Sensation of Chronic Pain, in the *Addiction-Free Pain Manage-*

ment Workbook offers an assessment tool to determine the level and intensity of both your psychological and physiologi-

> ## Goals for Process One, Part 2
>
> - Building a Pain Vocabulary
> - Determining Pain vs. Suffering

cal symptoms.

The purpose of this exercise is twofold: to help you build a vocabulary for talking about your pain, and to explore your reactions to your pain in order to determine whether your condition is more physiological or psychological—pain versus suffering.

Look at the chart that describes the types of pain you may experience. Notice that the chart has three columns and twenty rows. Each row contains three words that describe a certain symptom of pain. As you move from column one to column two to column three the words reflect an increasing intensity of that symptom of pain. The instructions ask you to circle the

> ### Items 1 to 8 are physical symptoms.
> ### Items 9 to 20 are emotional or psychological symptoms.

word(s) in each row that apply to you.

As you read through each set of descriptions you will circle the word(s) that describe your sensations and the number (on a scale of 0 to 10, with 0 meaning it's not very bad at all to 10 meaning it's very bad) that best describes the intensity of your

> ### Even-numbered items are more intense.

pain on a bad pain day.

Another useful feature of this instrument is that the even-numbered rows describe a more intense level of symptoms than the odd-numbered rows. You can look at the finished exercise and often determine very quickly whether your condition is more physically or psychologically based.

This instrument shown below gives you an increased vocabulary and insight to help you communicate accurately about your symptoms. This exercise also shows you that there is a difference between physically-based symptoms and psychologically-based pain symptoms. At the same time it gives you a deeper awareness of the issues that could impact successful treatment.

The Pain Vocabulary

SYMPTOMS (SENSATION OF CHRONIC PAIN)			LEVEL
1. ACHING	THROBBING	PULSING	
2. SPLITTING	PIERCING	POUNDING	
3. IRRITATED	SORE	SENSITIVE	
4. BURNING	STINGING	LACERATING	
5. TENDER	PAINFUL	HURTFUL	
6. INFLAMED	SHARP	SWOLLEN	
7. HOT	RADIATING	SPREADING	
8. TEARING	WRENCHING	SLASHING	
9. IRRITATING	NAGGING	DISTURBING	
10. DREADFUL	SEVERE	AWFUL	
11. TIRING	UPSETTING	AGGRAVATING	
12. DISTRESSING	EXCRUCIATING	AGONIZING	
13. UNCOMFORTABLE	TROUBLESOME	PROBLEMATIC	
14. TORTURING	GRUELING	EXHAUSTING	
15. WORRISOME	SADDENING	DEPRESSING	
16. FRIGHTENING	TERRIFYING	DREADFUL	
17. ANNOYING	TROUBLING	DISTURBING	
18. EXHAUSTING	FATIGUING	DEBILITATING	
19. FLEETING	BRIEF	MOMENTARY	
20. PERMANENT	CONSTANT	CEASELESS	

When using this Pain Vocabulary worksheet it's helpful to add up all of the scores for the physical pain indicators (rows 1–8) and for all the psychological pain indicators (rows 9–20) to see if the pain is predominately physical or psychological. You then need to add up the scores for the odd-numbered rows (1, 3, 5, etc.), which are indicators of less intense pain, and the even-numbered rows (2, 4, 6, etc.), which are indicators of more severe pain.

When you see how Donna and Matt completed this exercise below, notice that I have added additional *scoring* rows to help clarify the scoring process. Let's look at the results of Donna and Matt's exercise to see what you can learn.

Let's start by looking at how Matt completed the exercise for Process One, Part 2: The Biopsychosocial Sensation of Chronic Pain. The symptoms he circled are shown in the table below in **bold/underlined** and the level (or rating) is at the end under "Level."

Symptoms (Sensation of Chronic Pain)			Level
Physical Symptoms			
1. Aching	**Throbbing**	**Pulsing**	8
2. **Splitting**	**Piercing**	Pounding	7
3. **Irritated**	**Sore**	**Sensitive**	2
4. **Burning**	**Stinging**	**Lacerating**	8
5. Tender	**Painful**	**Hurtful**	8
6. Inflamed	**Sharp**	Swollen	7
7. **Hot**	**Radiating**	Spreading	9
8. Tearing	Wrenching	**Slashing**	8
Odd Subtotal = 27 Even Subtotal = 30 Physical Total = 57			
Psychological Symptoms			
9. **Irritating**	**Nagging**	**Disturbing**	8
10. **Dreadful**	**Severe**	**Awful**	10
11. **Tiring**	**Upsetting**	**Aggravating**	8

12.	DISTRESSING	EXCRUCIATING	AGONIZING	10
13.	UNCOMFORTABLE	TROUBLESOME	PROBLEMATIC	8
14.	TORTURING	GRUELING	EXHAUSTING	10
15.	WORRISOME	SADDENING	DEPRESSING	7
16.	FRIGHTENING	TERRIFYING	DREADFUL	8
17.	ANNOYING	TROUBLING	DISTURBING	8
18.	EXHAUSTING	FATIGUING	DEBILITATING	10
19.	FLEETING	BRIEF	MOMENTARY	3
20.	PERMANENT	CONSTANT	CEASELESS	10

ODD SUBTOTAL = 42	EVEN SUBTOTAL = 58	PSYCHOLOGICAL TOTAL = 100

ODD TOTAL = 69	EVEN TOTAL = 88	SYMPTOM TOTAL = 157

Matt's Sensations of Chronic Pain

Several points stand out when viewing Matt's completed exercise. The first impression is that he circled the majority of the items and at least one word was chosen in each row. At first glance his choices may seem to be fairly balanced between physiological and psychological. However, when looking closer you will notice that overall, the even-numbered rows scored higher than the odd (88 to 69), and the psychological symptoms (rows 9 to 20) had higher scores (100 to 57) than the physical symptoms (rows 1 to 8).

Even after deducting 20 points from the psychological category to balance the two separate categories to have the same possible total, Matt still scores 80 in the psychological category to 57 in the physical.

This information combined with the results of upcoming exercises gives you and your counselor or therapist insight into effective treatment planning. The results of Matt's exercise also show an early indication of the need to be aware of other problems.

Now let's review Donna's answers for the same exercise.

SYMPTOMS (SENSATION OF CHRONIC PAIN)			LEVEL
PHYSICAL SYMPTOMS			
1. ACHING	THROBBING	PULSING	0
2. SPLITTING	**PIERCING**	POUNDING	9
3. IRRITATED	SORE	SENSITIVE	0
4. **BURNING**	STINGING	**LACERATING**	9
5. TENDER	PAINFUL	HURTFUL	0
6. INFLAMED	**SHARP**	SWOLLEN	9
7. HOT	**RADIATING**	SPREADING	6
8. TEARING	WRENCHING	**SLASHING**	9

ODD SUBTOTAL = 6   EVEN SUBTOTAL = 36   PHYSICAL TOTAL = 42

PSYCHOLOGICAL SYMPTOMS			
9. IRRITATING	**NAGGING**	**DISTURBING**	10
10. DREADFUL	**SEVERE**	AWFUL	10
11. **TIRING**	UPSETTING	**AGGRAVATING**	10
12. **DISTRESSING**	**EXCRUCIATING**	**AGONIZING**	10
13. UNCOMFORTABLE	TROUBLESOME	**PROBLEMATIC**	8
14. TORTURING	**GRUELING**	**EXHAUSTING**	10
15. WORRISOME	SADDENING	DEPRESSING	0
16. FRIGHTENING	**TERRIFYING**	DREADFUL	8
17. **ANNOYING**	TROUBLING	DISTURBING	10
18. **EXHAUSTING**	**FATIGUING**	DEBILITATING	10
19. FLEETING	BRIEF	MOMENTARY	0
20. PERMANENT	CONSTANT	**CEASELESS**	10

ODD SUBTOTAL = 38   EVEN SUBTOTAL = 58   PSYCHOLOGICAL TOTAL = 96

ODD TOTAL = 44   EVEN TOTAL = 94   SYMPTOM TOTAL = 138

Donna's Sensation of Chronic Pain

As with Matt, several points stand out when viewing Donna's completed exercise. The first impression is that she did not circle the majority of the items and she did not select all three words for any item number. In fact, for several of the items she did not circle any symptoms at all.

However, when looking closer her choices seem to indicate low to moderate physiological problems and significant psychological symptoms. Overall the even-numbered rows scored much higher than the odd (94 to 44), and the psychological symptoms (rows 9 to 20) had much higher scores (96 to 42) than the physical symptoms (rows 1 to 8). Even after deducting 20 points from the psychological category to balance the two separate categories, Donna still scores 76 in the psychological category to only 42 in the physical.

As with Matt's results, the details of Donna's exercise also give an early indication of the need to be aware of other problems.

Take a few minutes to complete this
exercise in your APM workbook.

Now that you have an increased vocabulary, the next process is designed to help you identify the psychosocial effect you experience from your pain. This is accomplished by identifying irrational thought processes that lead to uncomfortable emotions and self-defeating behaviors.

Process One, Part 3: Exploring Your TFUARs

The primary goal of "Exploring Your TFUARs" is
to see how irrational thinking leads to emotional
and social distress.

The acronym TFUAR means
T = Thoughts
F = Feelings
U = Urges
A = Actions
R = Reactions or Relationships
This exercise is designed to help you explore your irrational thinking or thinking errors that occur as a result of your chronic

pain condition. That thinking often leads to uncomfortable emotions, which trigger self-defeating urges, usually followed by self-destructive behaviors. The table lists the questions asked in this exercise.

Exploring Your TFUARs Exercise

When you experience pain your TFUARs (thinking, feelings, urges, actions, and reactions of others) often change. The purpose of this exercise is to explore your personal accounts in each of the above areas when you experience pain.

Thinking: Prolonged exposure to chronic pain leads to irrational thinking (thinking errors) and self-defeating decision making. Please list below three thinking problems that you've experienced as a result of your pain.

Feelings: Use the Feelings Chart below to describe how you tend to feel when you're experiencing chronic pain at its worst, and how intense each feeling is on a scale of 0 (lowest intensity) to 10 (highest intensity).

The Feelings Chart

❏ Strong   or   ❏ Weak
                              How strong is the feeling? (0–10) _____

❏ Safe   or   ❏ Threatened
                              How strong is the feeling? (0–10) _____

❏ Angry   or   ❏ Caring
                              How strong is the feeling? (0–10) _____

❏ Fulfilled   or   ❏ Frustrated
                              How strong is the feeling? (0–10) _____

❏ Happy   or   ❏ Sad
                              How strong is the feeling? (0–10) _____

❏ Connected   or   ❏ Lonely
                              How strong is the feeling? (0–10) _____

❏ Proud   or   ❏ Ashamed, Guilty
                              How strong is the feeling? (0–10) _____

Urges: What do you have an urge (or impulse) to do when you're experiencing chronic pain at its worst?

Actions: What do you usually do when you're experiencing chronic pain at its worst?

The purpose of this exercise is twofold. First, it gives you insight into your psychological and behavioral patterns. Second, it gives you a new way of looking at how your pain experience has a biopsychosocial affect.

For example, Matt identified his three irrational thinking patterns: (1) I don't deserve this; (2) I have to do whatever it takes to stop this; and (3) I won't use meds next time, but this time I really need relief. Matt tends to react in a **top-dog** (power) fashion. Donna, on the other hand, came up with three **underdog** (victim) statements: (1) I'm better off dead; (2) What did I do to deserve this? and (3) Why can't I get better?

Both Donna and Matt identified similar feelings: weak, angry, sad, lonely, threatened, and frustrated. Donna rated weak at level 10 while Matt rated it level 5. Donna rated sad at a level 8 and Matt rated it 4. Both rated anger and frustration at a level 10, and Donna rated ashamed a level 10 while Matt did not rate either proud or ashamed.

While Matt had an urge to use pain medication, Donna had an urge to commit suicide. Matt often used pain medications, and if none were available he would find other self-defeating ways to distract himself. Donna tended to cry or try to go to sleep to escape.

Both Donna and Matt tended to isolate, with Matt hiding his pain with a tough facade and Donna feeling too much shame and guilt to reach out. The result was isolation from their support networks, which is a common tendency for a person experiencing chronic pain.

Take a few minutes to complete this exercise in your APM workbook.

Process One, Part 4: Stress and Chronic Pain

When you are asked to give up your pain medication, it's an important early treatment strategy to learn alternative methods to manage your pain. As I mentioned earlier, you need to learn about the connection between stress levels and pain symptoms, and to understand that stress management can also decrease your suffering. It's also important to learn simple stress reduction techniques that can be practiced during your early recovery period.

Learning to Identify Stress Levels

For Donna these new tools provided hope that eventual freedom from the medication was possible, but it would be a difficult journey. Stress identification and reduction is an important tool for anyone recovering from chemical dependency and chronic pain.

When you are aware of your stress levels, you can then take action to reduce your stress, which in turn leads to a decrease in your pain symptoms. Below is a reproduction of Process One, Part 4 from the *Addiction-Free Pain Management Workbook*, which both Donna and Matt utilized early in their treatment process.

General Stress Levels

A. **Low Stress Level (stress score: 0–3)**
   - Very relaxed; vacation mode
   - Stress is managed well; no discomfort
   - No notable distress or dysfunction

B. **Moderate Stress Levels (stress score: 4–6)**
   - Higher stress levels; normal operating level, no distress
   - Stress managed poorly at times; some discomfort but no distress
   - Some notable distress but no dysfunction

C. **Severe Stress Levels (stress score: 7–10)**
   - Very high stress levels
   - Stress is usually managed poorly
   - Stress causes notable distress and dysfunction

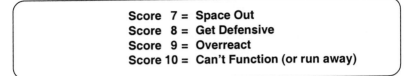

Score 7 = Space Out
Score 8 = Get Defensive
Score 9 = Overreact
Score 10 = Can't Function (or run away)

Learning to Measure Pain Levels

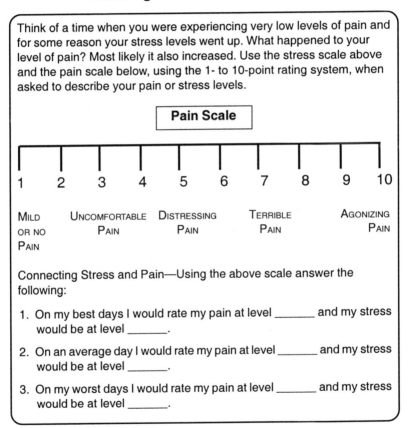

Think of a time when you were experiencing very low levels of pain and for some reason your stress levels went up. What happened to your level of pain? Most likely it also increased. Use the stress scale above and the pain scale below, using the 1- to 10-point rating system, when asked to describe your pain or stress levels.

Pain Scale

| 1 | 2 | 3 | 4 | 5 | 6 | 7 | 8 | 9 | 10 |

MILD OR NO PAIN — UNCOMFORTABLE PAIN — DISTRESSING PAIN — TERRIBLE PAIN — AGONIZING PAIN

Connecting Stress and Pain—Using the above scale answer the following:

1. On my best days I would rate my pain at level _____ and my stress would be at level _____.

2. On an average day I would rate my pain at level _____ and my stress would be at level _____.

3. On my worst days I would rate my pain at level _____ and my stress would be at level _____.

You are asked to use these charts to rate your pain and stress on your best days, on an average day, and on your worst pain day. The goal of this exercise is to help you see that pain and stress are connected and that good stress management can often reduce the intensity of pain.

> ## Primary Goal
>
> To show you the connection between stress and your pain

Both Donna and Matt were quickly able to see the connection between their stress and pain levels, and use these scales throughout the remainder of their treatment.

> ### Take a few minutes to complete this exercise in your APM workbook.

Once you are able to describe your pain symptoms and understand the biopsychosocial affects, the next task is to explore your use of pain medication. Prescription medication and other drugs (including alcohol) change how your brain and nervous system work. They either slow down, speed up, block out, change, or "blow up" (amplify) the messages and feelings that are generated by your brain. These drug effects make you feel different for a little while, but they don't actually change anything in the real world. They mask the chronic pain and change how you think, feel, and act but usually they don't make your life any better—instead, they often make life worse.

In the next chapter you will see how Donna and Matt completed Process Two from the APM workbook. It describes the biopsychosocial effects of medication and how the APM approach teaches you to make appropriate decisions regarding the use of your medication.

Chapter Six

The Effects of Medication and/or Other Drugs

Pain Relief vs. Euphoria

Some people with chronic pain who use potentially addictive medication for pain management never experience negative consequences. So why do other people develop an addictive disorder? In chapter two I discussed the addictive disorder process that occurs. For your review, I have reproduced the table of ten addictive disorder symptoms and will discuss the role euphoria plays.

1. Euphoria	6. Inability to Abstain
2. Craving	7. Addiction-Centered Lifestyle
3. Tolerance	8. Addictive Lifestyle Losses
4. Loss of Control	9. Continued Use Despite Problems
5. Withdrawal	10. Substance-Induced Organic Mental Disorders

As you saw earlier, Matt was finally able to break through his denial and admit that he often used his pain medication for its *euphoric effects*. This is a common realization for many people who experience problems managing their chronic pain. It's important to explore this a little further, using the information from the Gorski-CENAPS® Biopsychosocial Model of Alcoholism and Drug Addiction.

The Role Euphoria Plays

So why is there a transition from using pain medication for relief to using it for its euphoric effects? This question can be answered, in part, by understanding the relationship between brain reward mechanisms and the behavior of using psycho-active medication, or alcohol and other drugs. This demonstrates that the tendency toward *drug*-seeking behavior is strongly linked to progressive alterations in the function of your brain, and in late stages to the development of structural damage to your brain and other organ systems.

Research by the National Institute on Alcohol Abuse and Alcoholism (NIAAA) clearly shows that there are biomedical processes that occur within the brain that reinforces the regular and heavy use of psychoactive chemicals. These biomedical brain reinforcement processes are different from the classic withdrawal syndrome. The following is a summary of the research reported in the Alcohol Alert from NIAAA for July 1996.

The Biomedical Brain Reinforcement Process

- People will tend to repeat an action that brings pleasure or reward. The pleasure or reward provided by that action is called *positive reinforcement* or *euphoria*.
- Certain behaviors, especially those associated with survival needs, are linked to biochemical processes within the brain that cause powerful *biological reinforcement* for these behaviors.
- This biological reinforcement is related to the release of specific brain chemicals when the behavior is performed. These brain chemicals produce a sense of pleasure or reward.
- Alcohol and Other Drugs of Abuse (AOD's), including pain medication, produce chemicals that are surrogates of the naturally occurring brain chemicals that produce biological reinforcement.
- As a result the use of psychoactive chemicals causes a rewarding mental state (euphoria) that positively reinforces the initial use of the drugs. This rewarding mental state is defined as euphoria (euphoria is a state that is separate and distinct from the symptoms of intoxication).
- As a result individuals who receive positive reinforcement from drug use because of the production of these brain chemicals are more likely to engage in drug-seeking behavior and to use drugs regularly and heavily.
- The biochemical reinforcement that results from alcohol and other drug use is more powerful and persistently reinforcing than the biomedical reinforcement provided by other survival-related actions.

- As a result, people who experience this are more likely to feel that the use of alcohol and other drugs is more important than engaging in other vital survival-linked behaviors. As a result they will tend to use drugs instead of actively meeting other vital needs.
- This perception that alcohol and other drug use is more important than meeting other survival needs results in *drug-seeking behavior.*
- After drug-seeking behavior has been established, the brain undergoes certain *adaptive changes* to continue functioning despite the presence of the chemicals. This adaptation is called *tolerance.*
- Once this tolerance is established, further abnormalities occur in the brain when the drug is removed. In other words, the brain loses its capacity to function normally when drugs are not present.
- This low-grade abstinence-based brain dysfunction is distinct and different from the traditional acute withdrawal syndromes.
- This low-grade abstinence-based brain dysfunction is marked by feelings of discomfort, cravings, and difficulty finding gratification from other behaviors.
- This creates a desire to avoid the unpleasant sensations that occur in abstinence. This desire to avoid painful stimuli is called *negative reinforcement.*
- People who experience biological reinforcement (both positive and negative) are more likely to use drugs regularly and heavily.
- People who use drugs regularly and heavily are more likely to develop
  - physical dependence syndromes marked by tolerance and classic withdrawal symptoms; and
  - biomedical complications resulting from alcohol and drug use.
- There is evidence that people who are genetically susceptible and exposed prenatally to addiction may have pathological brain reward mechanisms.
- This pathological brain reward mechanism is marked by a below average release of packets of brain reward chemicals when not using the drug of choice.
  - When the drug of choice is used the brain releases abnormally large amounts of brain reward chemicals.
  - When not using, the person experiences a sense of anhedonia that is marked by a low-grade agitated depression and the inability to experience pleasure.
  - This feeling creates a craving for something, anything, that will relive the feeling.
- When the person finds the drug of choice that releases large amounts of brain reward chemicals, the person experiences a powerful sense of pleasure or euphoria. The experience feels so good that the patient begins seeking that experience.

This biomedical condition leads to psychological and social reinforcement.

Psychological Reinforcement

Your mind is capable of formulating thoughts that produce strong, positive, biological reinforcement. These thoughts often take the form of positive judgments about behavior that reflects itself in self-talk such as "Doing this is good for me!"

Positive judgments about behavior can be reinforcing of and by themselves because they are capable of activating the release of the biologically reinforcing brain chemicals. Positive judgment is said to *trigger* the state of reinforcement when this occurs.

When the biologically reinforcing brain chemicals are automatically released in response to a behavior, you feel pleasure and are more likely to judge the behavior as positive, which will stimulate the additional release of more, positively reinforcing brain chemicals. When this takes place the judgment is said to *enhance* the state of reinforcement.

Psychological Reinforcement=Gratification

Social Reinforcement

Social reinforcement occurs when the behaviors of others or the response of the environment is judged to be positive. These positive judgments about how people and the environment respond to you can trigger or enhance biological reinforcement.

Social Reinforcement=Reward

When you have an addictive disorder and need to use the APM *Medication Management Components,* special precautions are advised. It is important to know how to determine if you are using the medication appropriately.

That is why I developed the Pain Medication Recovery and Relapse Indicators, noted in the chart below. Using this checklist, combined with the Process Two exercises from the *Addiction-Free Pain Management Workbook*, gives you and your health-care providers a better chance of avoiding potential problems.

Pain Medication Recovery and Relapse Indicators

Recovery Indicators	Relapse Indicators
1. I am using medication as prescribed and in accordance with my Medication Management Treatment Plan.	1. I am not not using medication as prescribed, nor is it in accordance with my Medication Management Treatment Plan.
2. I am using pain medication only for its analgesic pain relief.	2. I am using pain medication for its euphoric effects and/or for its emotional management properties.
3. I am not experiencing obsession for or intrusive thoughts about the medication.	3. I am experiencing obsession for and/or intrusive thoughts about the medication.
4. I am not experiencing compulsion to use the medication inappropriately.	4. I am experiencing compulsion to use the medication.
5. I am not experiencing a craving to use the medication inappropriately.	5. I am experiencing a craving to use the medication.
6. I am not experiencing a loss of control of the medication.	6. I am experiencing a loss of control of the medication.
7. I am not experiencing intoxication from using the medication.	7. I am experiencing intoxication from using the medication.
8. I am not experiencing negative consequences from using the medication.	8. I am experiencing negative consequences from using the medication.
9. I am not experiencing any secondary related problems due to using the medication.	9. I am experiencing secondary related problems due to using the medication.
10. I am not experiencing a pain rebound effect from using the medication.	10. I am experiencing a pain rebound effect from using the medication.

Expectations vs. Reality

Process Two, Part 1: What You Wanted and What You Got

The first exercise in Process Two, Effects of Prescription and/or Other Drugs, asked you to list the type(s), amount(s), and frequency of the medication(s) you are currently using (or have used) to manage your pain. Don't forget to include alcohol because many people with chronic pain often use alcohol to help manage their pain.

You then explore what you wanted the drugs to do, the effects the drugs actually produced that made you believe you were getting what you wanted, and, finally, what you learned from completing the exercise.

> Take a few minutes to complete this
> exercise in your APM workbook.

At this point it would be extremely beneficial to share this information with your counselor or therapist as well as your primary physician and if that doctor is not certified in addiction medicine, you should consult someone with that training.

> Remember—Teamwork Is a Must!

The second exercise in Process Two explores some of the most common side effects and problems experienced from using pain medication. Prescription medication and other drugs (including alcohol) can seem to work for pain management in some instances. However, they often have serious physical side effects and/or lead to psychological and social problems.

Process Two, Part 2: Side Effects and Problems

Some of the most common problematic effects are listed below. You are asked to indicate how each applies to you, rating the degree of impact on you by circling the appropriate number (on a scale of 1 to 10, with 1 being not a problem to 10 being extremely problematic). After reviewing the effects listed below, I will describe how Donna and Matt completed this exercise.

Effects of Substances

1. INCREASED TOLERANCE (NEEDING MORE OF THE DRUG)

2. NAUSEA AND/OR VOMITING

3. FEELING SLEEPY, FATIGUED, OR DROWSY

4. BECOMING SHORT-TEMPERED (EASILY ANGERED)

5. IMPAIRED LIVER FUNCTIONS

6. ABDOMINAL PAIN OR CRAMPING

7. FEELING DOWN OR DEPRESSED

8. THOUGHTS OF SUICIDE

9. DECREASED SEXUALITY OR LIBIDO

10. INCREASED ANXIETY

11. INCREASED FAMILY OR RELATIONSHIP PROBLEMS

12. EUPHORIA—FEELING HIGH (INTOXICATED)

13. BECOMING CONFUSED OR DISORIENTED

14. BLURRED AND/OR DOUBLE VISION

15. STOMACH PAIN AND/OR ULCERS

16. BEING DEPENDENT/ADDICTED

17. URINE RETENTION

18. DIARRHEA

19. DECREASED JOB PERFORMANCE

20. DIFFICULTY HAVING FUN OR EXPERIENCING PLEASURE

Donna's Effects of Substances Exercise

EFFECTS OF SUBSTANCES	LEVEL
1. INCREASED TOLERANCE (NEEDING MORE OF THE DRUG)	9
2. NAUSEA AND/OR VOMITING	2
3. FEELING SLEEPY, FATIGUED, OR DROWSY	4
4. BECOMING SHORT-TEMPERED (EASILY ANGERED)	8
5. IMPAIRED LIVER FUNCTIONS	2
6. ABDOMINAL PAIN OR CRAMPING	4
7. FEELING DOWN OR DEPRESSED	8
8. THOUGHTS OF SUICIDE	3
9. DECREASED SEXUALITY OR LIBIDO	9
10. INCREASED ANXIETY	10
11. INCREASED FAMILY OR RELATIONSHIP PROBLEMS	8
12. EUPHORIA—FEELING HIGH (INTOXICATED)	8
13. BECOMING CONFUSED OR DISORIENTED	8
14. BLURRED AND/OR DOUBLE VISION	1
15. STOMACH PAIN AND/OR ULCERS	4
16. BEING DEPENDENT/ADDICTED	10
17. URINE RETENTION	1
18. DIARRHEA	1
19. DECREASED JOB PERFORMANCE	8
20. DIFFICULTY HAVING FUN OR EXPERIENCING PLEASURE	9

On her first attempt to complete this exercise, Donna had greatly underrated many of the symptoms. As she processed the results during session, she began to see how much she minimized the negative consequences and only focused on the benefits of using her medication.

Donna's second attempt was much more honest and showed an increase in most of the categories (listed above).

This exercise also opened up the discussion about other ways that her use of pain medication was negatively impacting her life, as well as being problematic for her family and friends. Now let's look at how Matt completed this exercise.

Matt's Effects of Substances Exercise

EFFECTS OF SUBSTANCES	LEVEL
1. INCREASED TOLERANCE (NEEDING MORE OF THE DRUG)	8
2. NAUSEA AND/OR VOMITING	2
3. FEELING SLEEPY, FATIGUED, OR DROWSY	3
4. BECOMING SHORT-TEMPERED (EASILY ANGERED)	9
5. IMPAIRED LIVER FUNCTIONS	2
6. ABDOMINAL PAIN OR CRAMPING	2
7. FEELING DOWN OR DEPRESSED	10
8. THOUGHTS OF SUICIDE	4
9. DECREASED SEXUALITY OR LIBIDO	10
10. INCREASED ANXIETY	10
11. INCREASED FAMILY OR RELATIONSHIP PROBLEMS	10
12. EUPHORIA—FEELING HIGH (INTOXICATED)	8
13. BECOMING CONFUSED OR DISORIENTED	9
14. BLURRED AND/OR DOUBLE VISION	1
15. STOMACH PAIN AND/OR ULCERS	3
16. BEING DEPENDENT/ADDICTED	10
17. URINE RETENTION	2
18. DIARRHEA	2
19. DECREASED JOB PERFORMANCE	10
20. DIFFICULTY HAVING FUN OR EXPERIENCING PLEASURE	10

Matt was very honest with his evaluation and reported that seeing all these negative side effects in one place was painful for him. He also noted that this realization had never stopped him from using before, but now he wanted to learn how to use this information to increase his positive self-talk. Again it was the processing of the exercise with someone else that had the most impact—not just filling out the forms.

> Take a few minutes to complete this exercise in your APM workbook.

Another common side effect for someone coping with chronic pain is depression. In addition, the medication and/or withdrawal from medication can also lead to clinical symptoms of depression. This is another area where teamwork is essential. If you are depressed you need to seek help from someone who specializes in identifying and treating depression.

You should also evaluate your grief and loss issues. A major part of the healing process for most people with chronic pain is identifying and grieving the loss of the healthy self, and/or prior level of functioning. In later chapters you will see how Donna and Matt addressed these issues.

> It is very important to uncover your beliefs about pain, as well as the benefits and disadvantages you experienced from taking your pain medication.

The next step in the assessment process is determining your beliefs about pain medication, your earliest experiences around pain and medication, and your perceived benefits and disadvantages of using your pain medication.

Process Three in the *Addiction-Free Pain Management Workbook* is a series of four decision-making exercises, which are designed to assist the chemical dependency/abuse assessment process. The first exercise explores your personal beliefs about pain and medication.

Process Three, Part 1: Personal Beliefs about Pain and Medication

Often your decision to use pain medication has been made because a doctor prescribed it, usually after a very brief consultation with you. Many doctors have minimal training in addictive disorders and may not be aware of the risks for some of their patients. On the other hand, some people mislead their doctors (intentionally or unintentionally), by not giving them an accurate picture of their past history with alcohol or other drug problems. Other factors in medication decision making center on your response to and beliefs about your pain.

In this exercise you are asked to refer back to Process One, Part 2 (Biopsychosocial Sensation...) and look at some of the words you circled that describe your pain on a bad day. Then review Process One, Part 3 (Exploring Your TFUARs) focusing on your three irrational thinking problems (thinking errors).

The experience of the pain sensations coupled with the strength of your thought process will often compel you to seek immediate pain relief without taking time to consider the possible negative consequences. You just want the pain to stop.

People who manage their pain effectively also want their pain to stop. However, recovery (abstinence and effective pain management) requires accurate self-monitoring, honest self-evaluation, and healthy self-change.

Prerequisites of APM Recovery

- Honest Self-Evaluation
- Accurate Self-Monitoring
- Healthy Self-Changing Behavior

The purpose of this exercise is for you to explore how you make decisions, so you can begin to make accurate, honest, and healthy choices about pain management and the way you use your pain medication.

You are asked to think back to the first time you took any medication (including alcohol) for pain relief and write about it like a story with a beginning, middle, and end. You are told to make sure to include the following:

- Your age at the time
- What you were doing
- Who you were with
- What happened to cause your pain
- What you were thinking about your pain
- How you were affected (or feelings produced) by your pain
- Who suggested the pain medication
- What it was, and how much you used

You are then asked what you wanted the medication to do for you and what you wanted the medication to help you cope with or escape from.

Ask Yourself

- What do you want the pain medication to do for you?
- Did you get what you wanted?

Both Donna and Matt experienced several useful insights after completing this exercise. Donna was able to see how her father frequently pushed pills at her when she complained about even mild symptoms. As a consequence, Donna learned from a very young age that pain was to be medicated, not tolerated.

Matt learned that pain must be hidden, not expressed. He remembers being shamed and humiliated by his father when he cried after spraining his ankle at age five. This set up his pattern for self-medicating and then hiding that he was doing so from others.

Take a few minutes to complete this exercise in your APM workbook.

Process Three, Part 2: Pain Medication Problem Checklist

The next step is to determine the risk or level of a potential addictive disorder (substance abuse or dependency). This is facilitated by Process Three, Part 2: The Pain Medication Problem Checklist.

Denial is one of the major symptoms of an addictive disorder, but in the case of someone addicted to prescribed pain medication for a "legitimate" reason the denial system is even more difficult to overcome. The Pain Medication Problem Checklist is designed to help you work around that resistance and denial, but this is only possible by your willingness to answer the questions honestly.

This instrument includes fifty "yes or no" questions using the addictive disorder criteria covered earlier, as well as the DSM-IV diagnostic criteria for substance abuse and substance dependency. However, they are rewritten in a less clinical manner.

Pain Medication Problem Checklist

1. Do you ever take medication in a larger dose than is prescribed by your doctor?
2. Do you ever take the medication more frequently than prescribed by your doctor?
3. Do you ever mix other drugs (including alcohol) with your prescribed medication without your doctor's knowledge or approval?
4. Do you sometimes use mood-altering drugs that have been prescribed for someone else?
5. Do you ever use any other drugs that aren't prescribed for you by your doctor? (These might be medicines like diet pills, sleep aids, stay-awake pills, or some of the herbal energy supplements that make you high or give you a buzz.)
6. When you're using pain medication (including alcohol) and other drugs, do you ever put yourself in situations that raise your risk of getting hurt, having problems, or hurting others? (This includes things like driving while using prescriptions, alcohol, or other drugs; having sex without protection; getting into fights; skipping work; committing crimes; etc.)
7. Have you ever realized that you need to take more medication than you used to in order to get the pain relief you desire?

---

8. If you use the same amount of medication all the time, do you experience a reduction in your pain relief or are you tempted to increase the dose?

9. Have you ever been ashamed of your behavior while under the influence of your pain medication or of something that happened while you were taking it?

10. Have you ever felt sick or anxious (or experienced other withdrawal symptoms) when you suddenly stopped using your medication?

11. Have you ever used your medication or other drugs (including alcohol) to avoid withdrawal symptoms?

12. Have you ever hidden from (or not told) one doctor what you have been given by another doctor (or about use of over-the-counter medication)?

13. Have you ever done things while you were using pain medication (including alcohol) and other drugs that you regretted or that made you feel guilty or ashamed?

14. Have you had a persistent desire or made unsuccessful efforts to cut down or control your medication?

15. Have you ever used your medication (including alcohol) or other drugs to try to escape from or cope with a problem or situation that you didn't know any other way to deal with?

16. Do you use other drugs (including alcohol) when not taking your medication?

17. Do you spend a great deal of your time seeing several doctors (doctor shopping), being under the influence, or recovering from the effects of your medication?

18. Has anyone else (a spouse, parent, brother, sister, boss, or friend) ever told you that they thought you might have a problem with your prescription drug use?

19. Have you continued to use your medication despite having persistent or frequent physical or psychological problems caused by the medication (for example, impaired liver functions or depression)?

20. Have you ever experienced legal problems due to substance-related issues (such as forging prescriptions or driving while taking your mood-altering medication)?

21. Have you ever used pain medication without really needing it for physical pain?

22. Have you ever used pain medication (including alcohol) to cope with uncomfortable feelings or to manage stress?

23. Have you ever thought that you might have a problem with your prescription drug use?

24. Have you ever failed to finish home or work commitments because you were using pain medication (including alcohol) or drugs or were in withdrawal?

25. Have you ever seen a counselor or other professional for help about your prescription drug (or alcohol and/or other drug) use?

26. Have you ever used more medication or used over a longer period of time than you originally intended?

27. Have you ever let other people down whom you cared about because you were using pain medication (including alcohol) or drugs or were in withdrawal?

28. Have your family, employer, coworkers, or friends ever been annoyed by or criticized you because of your use of pain medication (including alcohol)?

29. Have your family or friends ever been concerned about the amount or frequency of the pain medication you take (including alcohol)?

30. Have you had arguments with your spouse or family members because of something that happened when you were using pain medication?

31. Have you ever been too sick to go to work as a result of using pain medications (including alcohol) or other drugs? (This includes bad hangovers or withdrawal.)

32. Have you ever had problems with friends as a result of your use of pain medication (including alcohol) or other drugs?

33. Have you ever gotten physically sick as a result of taking your pain medication (including alcohol) or other drugs?

34. Have you ever continued using pain medication (including alcohol) or drugs even though you knew they were causing problems or making your problems worse?

35. Has a doctor or counselor ever told you that he or she thought you had a serious problem with pain medication (including alcohol) or other drugs?

36. Have you ever been a patient in a mental health clinic or hospital where using pain medication was at least a part of your problem?

37. Have you noticed a decrease in experiencing fun or pleasure as a result of taking the pain medication or recovering from its effects?

38. Have you experienced depression or even thoughts of suicide while taking pain medication?

39. Do you ever feel guilty or ashamed for taking pain medication?

40. Have you ever experienced the inability to remember events or blocks of time while under the influence of pain medication?

41. Have you ever attended any self-help meetings to deal with pain medication or problems that occurred, at least in part, because you were taking the medication?

42. Have you ever been in a hospital as a direct (or indirect) result of taking pain medication?
43. Do you ever use your medication to feel high (euphoria)?
44. If you were told you had to stop your pain medication because of a medical problem would it be difficult for you to stop?
45. Have you ever lied to or mislead a doctor in order to receive more (or stronger) pain medication?
46. Have you ever done anything that violated your morals or values as a result of being under the influence of pain medication (including alcohol) or other drugs?
47. Have you lost contact with your spirituality (or religious beliefs) while taking pain medication (including alcohol) or other drugs?
48. Do you feel deprived or even angry when you can't get your pain medication as quickly as you would like (or get enough of your pain medication)?
49. Do you ever find yourself making excuses to use more medication than was prescribed by your doctor?
50. Did you feel uncomfortable or have the urge to lie (or rationalize/ minimize) when answering any of the above questions?

Process Three, Part 3: Interpreting the Pain Medication Problem Checklist

The interpretation of the checklist follows in Part Three, asking you to score the number of "yes" answers, then check your level or risk of addiction.

- **Low risk of addiction:** if you answered "no" to all the questions.
- **High risk of addiction (substance abuse):** if you answer "yes" to three or more of questions 1 to 20 and "no" to the remaining questions.
- **Early-stage addiction (substance dependency):** if you have three or more "yes" answers to questions 1 to 20 and between three to six "yes" answers for the remainder of the questions.
- **Middle-stage addiction:** if you have three or more "yes" answers to questions 1 to 20 and between seven and ten "yes" answers to the remainder of the questions.
- **Late-stage addiction:** if there are three or more "yes" answers to questions 1 to 20 and eleven or more "yes" answers to the remaining questions.

You are then asked if you agree that the result of the Pain Medication Problem Checklist accurately describes your current risk or level of addiction. Donna and Matt both saw themselves in late-stage addiction before completing this exercise, and the results of their checklists validated their impressions.

The discussion that follows this exercise is much more important than the exercise itself and you should share this with your counselor or therapist and/or other trusted team members. This process helps you see clearly some of the problems you may have as a direct result of chemical use. Even though Donna and Matt were not in denial about the seriousness of their addiction, they were both surprised about the extensive effect of their drug use.

> Take a few minutes to complete this
> exercise in your APM workbook.

Process Three, Part 4: The Decision to Stop

This final part of the Process Three exercises has you list both the benefits and disadvantages of using your pain medication by completing the following form. The final question asks you whether you think the benefits you expected from your medication were worth the pain and problems that you experienced.

Benefits: List the main things that were better for you because you used pain medication (including alcohol and other drugs).	**Disadvantages:** List the main things that were worse for you, or problems that you had because you used pain medication (including alcohol and other drugs).

Biopsychosocial History

The final part of a complete self-assessment includes a biopsychosocial and trauma history. Significant others and/or family members should be consulted when you're gathering this information because sometimes you might have forgotten or blocked out crucial information. Family-of-origin issues and other traumatic situations have a significant impact on treatment planning and treatment outcome, so your counselor or therapist needs to have the whole picture.

There are several instances in the pain literature that report chronic pain conditions can restimulate Post-traumatic Stress Disorders. This was certainly the case for Donna and to a slightly lesser degree for Matt as well. As you will see in later chapters this information makes a difference in treatment approaches.

> Assessments need to be ongoing throughout
> the APM treatment process.

It is also important to note that the identification and self-assessment process needs to continue throughout the entire treatment process. The APM system is designed to facilitate this ongoing assessment. The more you learn about yourself the more effective your recovery and pain management program becomes.

Process 4: Abstinence Contract and Intervention Planning

Another useful tool to help you avoid relapse early on is Process Four in the *Addiction-Free Pain Management Workbook*, which includes intervention planning and abstinence contracting.

Part 1-A of this process asks you to identify your current problems, listing how the problems are connected to your inappropriate use of pain medication, and asking for a commitment to stop. At this point you are also asked to identify a situation in the near future that could cause you to start using pain medication inappropriately.

Part 1-B gives you a chart to summarize the information. The intervention plan outlines your roles and the roles of the therapist/counselor and at least three significant others. This exercise is reproduced on page ___.

Both Donna and Matt had some difficulty in choosing appropriate significant others. It was also difficult for them to come up with effective intervention requests. After several attempts they were able to find supportive people who were willing and able to be a part of an effective relapse prevention network.

The other important parts of Process Four in the *Addiction-Free Pain Management Workbook* are the presenting-problem exercises and the abstinence contract. The Process Four exercises are shown here.

Process Four, Part 1–A: Presenting Problems

1. **Presenting problems:** What are the presenting problems that caused you to seek help at this time? (Why did you seek help now? Why not yesterday or next week? What would have happened if you didn't seek help now? What problems or negative consequences can this workbook help you to avoid?)

2. **Relationship to inappropriate use of pain medication:** How is each presenting problem related to your inappropriate use of pain medication and/or to an ineffective pain management program? How is this problem related to your inappropriate use of pain medication (including alcohol) or other mood-altering substances? Did the chemicals cause you to have this problem? (Would you have this problem if you never inappropriately used pain medication including alcohol or other drugs?) Did inappropriate use of pain medication (including alcohol) or other drugs make this problem worse than it would have been if you hadn't been using it?

3. **Consequences of not stopping:** What additional problems could you experience if you keep inappropriately using pain medication (including alcohol) or other drugs despite these problems? (What are the benefits? What are the disadvantages? What is the best thing that could happen? What is the worst? What is the most likely thing that will probably happen?)

---

4. **The Abstinence Commitment:** Are you willing to make a commitment not to inappropriately use pain medication (including alcohol) or other drugs for [*name the specific period of time*:_____ _____]? (This should be done with the assistance of your doctor and counselor.) Explain your answer.

5. **Immediate high-risk situations:** Are you facing any situations in the near future that could cause you to inappropriately use pain medication (including alcohol) or other drugs despite your commitment not to? Explain your answer.

6. **The APM/RPC commitment:** Are you willing to make an agreement to complete the APM/RPC process in order to learn how to identify and manage those high-risk situations without inappropriately using pain medication (including alcohol) or other drugs?

❑ Yes   ❑ No   ❑ Unsure   Explain your answer.

Process Four, Part 1–B: Presenting Problem Report Form

My Presenting Problems	Relationship to Inappropriate Pain Medication (Including Alcohol) or Other Mood-Altering Drug Use	Consequences If I Keep Using

Process Four, Part 2: APM/RPC Abstinence Contract

I, _____, do
hereby agree to ABSTAIN from using any inappropriate pain medication (including alcohol) or other drugs and to continue an effective pain
management program while I am working on this APM/RPC Workbook.

Should I return to using inappropriate pain medication (including
alcohol) or other drugs and/or deviating from my pain management
program, I will immediately seek help from an appropriate treatment
professional. I will also be open to outpatient or residential inpatient
treatment if determined necessary by that treatment professional.

I also agree to submit to random drug screens at the discretion of the
treatment professional. Unwillingness to submit to a breath, blood, or
urine test will be interpreted as a clear indicator that I have been using
mood-altering chemicals or drinking alcohol and that I need immediate
intervention.

I will consult with _____ (an addiction
medicine practitioner/specialist) regarding any medications prescribed
to me by any physician. (Their phone number is: _____)

_____   _____
Signature   Date

_____   _____
Signature of Witness   Date

*This abstinence contract was adapted from the abstinence contract
developed and field tested by CENAPS® consultant and trainer, Tim
Dworniczek, ACRPS.*

Process Four, Part 3: Relapse Intervention Planning

Relapse Intervention Plan: One of the goals of completing this
workbook is to prepare you to quickly stop the inappropriate use of
pain medication (including alcohol) and other drugs, or ineffective pain
management, should it occur. This process is called developing a
relapse intervention plan.

Factors that stop relapse quickly: Your response to relapse will be
determined in large part by the following three factors: (1) what you were

told will happen if you start inappropriately using pain medication (including alcohol) or other drugs or start mismanaging your pain management program; (2) what you can do to stop using pain medication (including alcohol) or other drugs and/or get back to using an effective pain management program if relapse occurs; and (3) the approach of the treatment professionals who deal with you after the relapse has occurred.

Guidelines that stop relapse quickly should it occur. It's a mistaken belief that "If you take one dose of a drug you will lose control and not be able to stop until you hit bottom." There are two reasons *not* to believe this: First, it's not true. Many chemically dependent people have short-term and low-consequence relapses and get back into recovery before serious damage occurs. Second, this approach programs you for a long-term catastrophic relapse episode. If you do start to inappropriately use pain medication (including alcohol) or other drugs, the misleading voice may pop into your head saying, "If you take one dose of a drug you will lose control and not be able to stop until you hit bottom." You may then say to yourself, "Great, now I can keep medicating until I hit bottom." This does not mean it's perfectly fine to take single drug doses whenever the mood strikes or as long as your life doesn't fall apart. You still have to be vigilant. "Single dosing" is a high-risk situation. Fortunately, if you do start to inappropriately use pain medication (including alcohol) or other drugs, you will hit moments of sanity where you can choose to stop the relapse and get help. At these moments it is important to act immediately. If you wait, the urge to use again will come back and the opportunity will be lost. If you do start to inappropriately use pain medication including alcohol and other drugs and hit a moment of sanity where you want to stop, the four most effective things for you to do are:

• Read your prepared relapse intervention plan, which should always be readily accessible (you also should have given copies to significant others).

• Immediately stop using and get out of the situation that supports inappropriate use of pain medication (including alcohol) and other drugs.

• Immediately call for help and get into a sobriety supportive-situation.

• Call a counselor or sponsor, go to a treatment program, or get to a support-group meeting.

The Relapse Intervention Plan: In its simplest form, developing a relapse intervention plan consists of processing the following three questions by developing a specific written plan in response to each question.

1. What is the counselor supposed to do if you relapse, stop coming to sessions, or fail to honor your treatment or abstinence contract?

2. What are you going to do to get back into recovery if you start inappropriately using pain medication (including alcohol) or other drugs so that you can stop using before you hit bottom?

3. Who are three significant others who have an investment in your recovery, and what is each of them supposed to do if relapse occurs? Make sure you have their day and night phone numbers accessible, and that they have a copy of this plan.

A. Name of Significant Other #1: _____
   Phone: _____

   What are they supposed to do? _____

   _____

B. Name of Significant Other #2: _____
   Phone: _____

   What are they supposed to do? _____

   _____

C. Name of Significant Other #3: _____
   Phone: _____

   What are they supposed to do? _____

   _____

Managing Resistance and Denial

Going through the exercises above can increase your motivation and encourage you to be successful in your ongoing recovery process. These exercises are part of the Denial Management Counseling approach that will be described in the next chapter.

Both Donna and Matt had made numerous commitments to stop abusing their pain medications in the past, but this time they needed to put it in writing and sign their names to that commitment. Matt shared later that having this signed contract helped him avoid using on several occasions.

Connecting Cause and Effect

For Donna it was important to finally connect with the fact that many of the problems she was experiencing were directly connected to her use of pain medication. Once she realized what the problems were, she was more willing to make a commitment to stop using her old ways of behaving and learn safer ways of coping.

Take a few minutes to complete these exercises in your APM workbook.

Other early treatment approaches—*the Holistic Treatment Processes*—including non-psychoactive pain medication, physical therapy, hydrotherapy, non-pharmacological pain management, and chemical dependency education should be implemented when needed to facilitate your detoxification and stabilization. These are some of the treatment approaches that will be covered in the next chapter and are also crucial to have in place to facilitate your relapse intervention plan. It's important to remember that sometimes it is necessary to implement these interventions early on in your treatment process.

Chapter Seven

APM Holistic Treatment Processes

> ### Active vs. Passive

Earlier I discussed that the APM system is based on the concept that an active, multidimensional approach is required to obtain favorable treatment outcomes. Many chemical dependency treatment programs and pain clinics may try to put you in a passive role, which is counterproductive.

In addition to putting you in a passive role, some chronic pain treatments fall short because they lack a multidimensional approach. Chronic pain patients require an active, biopsychosocial approach to treatment; for example, the treatment plan might include exercises, chiropractic treatment, cognitive-behavioral strategies, and massage therapy.

For many of you part of this multidimensional approach would include helping you accept the necessity for recovery. This is where the CENAPS® Model of Denial Management Counseling (DMC) can be utilized.

Denial Management Counseling

Denial Management Counseling is a treatment modality designed to assist people with alcohol and drug-related problems who have high levels of denial and treatment resistance. Many of you may match these criteria. The DMC procedures focus on completing the *Denial Management Counseling Workbook* by Terence T. Gorski and Stephen F. Grinstead.

Goals of DMC

- Interrupt denial
- Increase recognition of addiction-related life problems
- Identify the real problems and losses from drug use
- Motivate you to accept referral to the next level of treatment

Holistic Treatment Approaches

The *Addiction-Free Pain Management Workbook* incorporates a portion of the DMC process by using an abstinence contract and the decision-making exercises that were explained earlier. Along with DMC, other treatment modalities need to be added at the same time to address the synergistic effects of the addictive disorder and the chronic pain disorder (i.e., the Addiction Pain Syndrome).

Massage Therapy and Physical Therapy

One early approach you might consider is massage therapy. When using massage therapy it's important to realize there will be some immediate pain relief and reduced muscle tension, but it will be short-lived if not followed with other measures. This is understandable because there are many precursors or triggers for muscle tension that often resurface soon after the massage session. Therefore, other measures must be implemented that are specific to your individual needs, and they must be used in the proper sequence.

Some of the methods that are successful in resolving these other precursors to pain are learning to use relaxation and meditation techniques, a customized exercise discipline, the use of biofeedback, and implementing a proper nutrition procedure, which is covered in a later chapter.

Using Physical Therapy with Hydrotherapy

Many health-care providers promote the combination of physical therapy and hydrotherapy to help you learn how to strengthen and recondition your body, thus becoming active participants in your healing.

Hydrotherapy and a water-based exercise program can be an extremely helpful, active modality for people with chronic pain. Because water buoys the body, the stress and strain is removed while in the water. Exercising in the water for short periods of time has benefits equal to several hours of land-based exercise, without some of the negative side affects.

Hydrotherapy and swimming were important components of Matt's pain management program, especially because land-based exercise tended to be problematic for him. In fact, over-exercising led Matt to seek relief with pain medication several times.

Biofeedback

Biofeedback has proven to be another effective, active method that you can learn to further participate in your own treatment.

The condition of dysponesis, also called faulty bracing, is where you tense up your muscles to pain thereby intensifying the pain experience. One of the most direct methods for coping with dysponesis involves the use of biofeedback. This procedure teaches you to let go of stress and tension.

An effective biofeedback training program should be progressive and include several steps. The program starts with an accurate diagnosis of your problem followed by implementation of the proper treatment modality and time for you to practice in situations that simulate instances in which the symptoms most often arise. Learning to use meditation and relaxation techniques to reduce stress is also a helpful complement to the biofeedback process.

Hypnosis and Meditation

Stress-reduction practice, as well as other holistic approaches, combined with biofeedback, has proven to be an excellent way to reduce pain symptoms. Hypnosis and meditation are effective *belief and attitude* therapy approaches that have proven successful in treating chronic pain.

> Hypnosis and medication have proven effective in chronic pain treatment.

Both Donna and Matt spent a portion of most of their psychotherapy sessions practicing some of these techniques.

The Emotional Link

Learning to identify and manage your uncomfortable or painful emotions is crucial for effective pain management and relapse prevention. In chapter nine you will look at a feeling checklist and be exposed to some feeling-management skills.

Most chemical dependency treatment professionals realize the importance of teaching you how to appropriately deal with your emotional issues to reduce your stress and anxiety. The CENAPS® model is based in part on the belief that avoiding painful emotions will often lead you to relapse.

It is unfortunate that many pain clinics do not focus on the emotional component of pain, as dealing with uncomfortable feelings is so important for effective pain management. In a review of thirty-two multi-modal pain treatment programs, many interventions and treatment approaches were being used; however, none of those programs used emotional management approaches.

It's important to have several different treatment strategies to deal with emotions such as anger, depression, and anxiety. Some of the methods include cognitive-behavioral therapy exercises, as well as meditation and relaxation techniques. It is also important to address the link between chronic pain and emotions, especially when there is clear and unambiguous evidence of suppressed or repressed emotional issues, where dynamic psychotherapy is an effective treatment modality.

> Using the Twelve Steps to Manage Pain

In her book *Living Well: A Twelve-Step Response to Chronic Illness and Disability,* Martha Cleveland maintains that dealing with the emotional component of chronic pain is an extremely effective treatment approach. Cleveland adapts and incorporates the Twelve Steps of Alcoholics Anonymous, showing people with chronic pain issues how to improve the quality of their lives and effectively deal with their emotions. Both Donna and Matt used Cleveland's book as part of their healing process.

Meditation

Dealing with emotions and promoting faster healing can be facilitated through the use of meditation. There is often misunderstanding about what meditation is and whether or not it's effective. However, there is substantial literature on the usefulness of meditation.

The practice of meditation can lead to true and lasting healing. Meditation takes on many diverse definitions for different individuals. For some, meditation is used for stress reduction; for others, it's a way of interconnecting parts of the brain; and still others find it helpful in healing the splits in personality and integrating wholeness.

The use of meditation can also be used for improving quality of life and for self-healing. Meditation is also a part of the Twelve-Step process—the Eleventh Step. Step Eleven shows people with chronic pain how to apply it to their healing process. You can learn how to effectively use the meditation portion of that step.

Dealing with Grief/Loss Issues

One of the most difficult and crucial emotional issues that needs resolution for successful recovery and effective pain management is healing the grief and loss of your physical condition and/or prior level of functioning.

Psychotherapists have experience facilitating the grieving process and should be part of your APM team. A review of the works of Elizabeth Kubler-Ross on the grieving process is also helpful in this regard.

Kubler-Ross Stages of Grieving

- Denial
- Anger
- Bargaining
- Depression
- Acceptance

Like Kubler-Ross I believe that grieving is important for healing. Working through the denial issues and moving into letting go of the anger is the starting point. Many people go through a pleading/bargaining phase by not being willing to accept the full reality of their condition. This often leads to profound sadness and depression.

Unlike Kubler-Ross I don't think that acceptance is the final stage of the grieving process. I believe the last stage is hope. What I mean by that is this: for ongoing recovery and effective pain management I believe you need to come to the realization that your life is great just the way it is. Knowing that, you can be a healthy, functioning human being—the hope and belief that your life can be better than ever before.

Grief work was an important part of healing for both Donna and Matt, but especially so for Matt. One of the reasons Matt used medication was to help him function at a higher level of physical activity. Unfortunately, he would often increase the severity of his pain because when he was under the influence of the pain medication he tended to overextend himself, and in some cases he actually experienced new injuries as a result of being impaired.

In addition, Matt had some serious shame issues regarding what defines a "real" man, especially in the area of sexuality. In fact, this sexuality/shame issue was the major precursor to his divorce, as well as his tendency to avoid new intimate relationships. For Matt, working through this grief/loss and shame was crucial to his avoiding future relapse episodes.

Acupuncture

As an alternative pain-reduction procedure, acupuncture needs to be briefly discussed. There are pros and cons of acupuncture. You need to look at both the positive aspects of many people gaining significant pain reduction and the fact that many people experience no benefit or limited benefit.

Of course, another drawback of this procedure is the danger of becoming a frequent acupuncture patient, leading you to possibly taking on a passive role in treatment, which is counterproductive to your effective, ongoing pain management.

Donna experienced no benefit from acupuncture, while Matt experienced only limited relief and discontinued it after a few sessions. Many of my other chronic pain patients, however, have experienced significant benefits from acupuncture.

> ## Chiropractic treatment is often effective.

Chiropractic Treatment

Many chronic pain patients receive long-term pain reduction when undergoing chiropractic treatment. Chiropractic adjustments restore proper motion and function to damaged joints, thereby reducing irritation to associated muscles and nerves.

Most chiropractors are trained in nutrition and many include dietary planning and nutrient supplementation in their treatment. This process helps to build up your immune system while at the same time raising your pain threshold. Later in this chapter I discuss the importance of using supplements as part of the healing process.

> ## Chiropractic care works for many chronic pain conditions.

There are a number of published studies supporting the effectiveness of chiropractic care for several types of chronic pain. For example, a study by Milne reported that out of 150 patients with migraine headaches, 98 percent experienced immediate relief of migraine through adjustments of the neck and through traction. Because many people are prescribed potentially addictive medication for migraine relief, chiropractic treatment could be a much safer, and often a more effective, alternative.

The largest comparative study on treatment of back pain (Meade) concluded that chiropractic care was the superior treatment for chronic low-back pain. Some case studies on whiplash treatment suggest that chiropractic care is effective for relieving the chronic pain often experienced after these injuries.

Activator Methods®
Chiropractic Technique

One of the newer, scientifically based chiropractic procedures is the Activator Methods® Chiropractic Technique. The Activator Methods® Chiropractic Technique (AMCT) is a process of analysis and instrumentation, which is designed to monitor and affect your neuromusculoskeletal system. This method evolved from more than twenty-five years of empirical study and ten years of clinical research. AMCT uses the latest advances in orthopedic, neurological, and chiropractic examinations to detect joint dysfunction in the spinal column and extremities for improved patient care. The implement that is used is the Activator Adjusting Instrument (AAI), which is a patented, hand-held adjusting device, designed to generate reproducible and controlled results.

However, this process requires chiropractors to become certified via examinations to ensure a level of proficiency needed for effective and safe outcomes. More than 31,000 doctors have been trained in AMCT and 2,500 doctors are proficiency rated, making AMCT the most widely used technique worldwide, a testament to its safety and efficacy. A certified chiropractor can be located by calling a referral service toll free at (800) 598-0224, or by visiting the Web site *www.Activator.com.*

From Surviving to Thriving

Because part of some people's preoccupation with medication stems from an appropriate need for pain reduction, non-pharmacological pain treatment modalities need to be developed and put into place. An important goal during this phase of treatment is to begin empowering yourself by relieving yourself of the passive role in dealing with your pain. You need to implement a proactive approach, including the above modalities and cognitive-behavioral strategies.

There are many other alternative nontraditional pain-management modalities that a trained treatment team can help you implement as indicated by your specific needs. These holistic treatment processes were covered earlier (see pages 130–137). All the chosen strategies can then become an integral part of your relapse prevention plan, which I will cover later.

APM uses an individualized and holistic
team approach.

An important point to consider is that the traditional "cookie-cutter" approach never did deliver positive treatment outcomes with the *usual* chemical dependency patient. Therefore, with the significant added issues of chronic pain (the addiction pain syndrome), the approaches used must be individualized as well as holistic. To that end, you must insist on teamwork among all your health-care providers. Remember that you are the captain of your team, but you need a coach and other players to win.

Nutrition and Healing

There appears to be a lack of information and a great deal of misinformation regarding the role of proper nutrition for pain management. The purpose of this section is to introduce you to some of the methods used as a part of the APM treatment approach.

The importance of proper diet and exercise as a part of addictive disorder recovery has been recognized for a long time. There is a significant amount of information about this in the recovery literature, such as the *books Passages Through Recovery* (Gorski) and *Staying Sober* (Gorski and Miller).

There is also substantial pain-management literature emphasizing the importance of nutrition and exercise in the healing process and effective pain management. In fact, Dr. Margaret Caudill devotes an entire chapter of her book, *Managing Pain Before it Manages You*, on the importance of nutrition in an effective pain management program.

Later on I will discuss and suggest some effective diet and exercise treatment plans and discuss the plans developed by Donna and Matt. Because in-depth coverage of nutrition and exercise is beyond the scope of this book, you will be introduced to several resources for additional information in the bibliography. You may also consider obtaining referrals to appropriate nutritionists in your area. Be sure your treatment providers have releases signed to facilitate teamwork, treatment planning, and effective follow-up.

Nutrition and Pain: Foods that Help or Hinder

Diet may have little effect on your experience of pain, but it probably influences the way you perceive your pain by the way it is associated with inflammation. Because the metabolization of some fats and fatty acids may have a tendency to intensify the inflammation response, you should closely monitor their intake. In addition, some foods tend to act as triggers for certain pain conditions, such as migraine headaches.

Some of the problem substances that are linked to increases in pain are caffeine, alcohol, monosodium glutamate (MSG), and aspartame (NutraSweet®). On the other hand, some foods have been credited with pain reduction. Dr. Caudill reports some foods linked to a decrease in pain include vegetarian diets as well as diets high in complex carbohydrates and low in protein.

The use of a **food diary** can be beneficial in discovering which foods are part of your problem and which are helpful. For optimal success this should be done under the supervision of a doctor or nutritionist.

Consumption of bioflavonoids, as found in fresh cherries, as well as eating other foods such as vegetables, legumes, whole grains, and some types of nuts can supplement some of the vitamins that appear to be deficient in people with chronic pain. However, caution must be used when taking vitamin and mineral supplements, especially with the tendency to use mega-doses. Two conditions that seem to respond well to dietary changes are rheumatoid arthritis and gout.

Proper nutrition plays an important role in the art of **naturopathy** (nature cure). The philosophy of naturopathic healing is based in part on the following:

- Discover and eliminate the primary cause of pain;
- use the most natural, nontoxic, and least invasive therapy possible;
- treat the whole person;
- teach the person to develop a healthy diet; and
- support the body's own healing abilities.

Recent studies provide significant information and scientific data to ensure the safety and effectiveness of some naturopathic remedies. However, some therapies using colonic irrigation may lead to unwanted side effects, such as infections.

Importance of Weight Management

Another important reason for good nutrition is weight management. Many chronic pain conditions are worsened by too much weight. If you also have a problem with overeating and/or excess weight you could benefit by completing *Food Addiction: The Recovery and Relapse Prevention Workbook,* by Stephen F. Grinstead and Terence T. Gorski.

Too much weight can lead to an increase in back pain and intensify the pressure on degenerative joints. Being underweight can also lead to problems of increased sickness and an impaired immune system. This is one of the reasons APM incorporates nutrition and exercise into every treatment plan.

> The human body functions most effectively at its optimal weight.

While Matt was at his optimal weight, Donna needed some extra interventions to help her reduce her weight by at least fifty pounds. The extra weight made it difficult for Donna to want to exercise, due to her fear of being judged by those watching her. In addition to a proper food plan (an integral part of her healthy living plan), the turning point for Donna was a prescription to join a hydrotherapy class that also catered to overweight patients. As she began to lose weight her pain started to decrease, while her self-esteem and motivation increased.

Herbal and Homeopathic Remedies

Some chronic pain practitioners use the pain-relieving effects of herbs as an adjunct to a healthy nutritional plan. According to the World Health Organization about 80 percent of the world uses herbal remedies.

For example, the science of herbs is at the core of traditional Chinese medicine. Also, a significant percentage of pharmaceutical products in the United States contain ingredients from plants. Fortunately, there has been an increase in research on herbal remedies, several of which have proven beneficial with negligible side effects.

On the other hand, some herbs have been found to have serious—and in some cases lethal—side effects. The vast majority of homeopathic medicines are also derived from plants, but before a remedy can be recognized as an official homeopathic medicine it must be tested scientifically on healthy humans under a double-blind procedure to determine safety and effectiveness.

Exercise and Healing

Most people will readily agree that regular exercise is good for you, and when combined with a healthy diet it will help people gain or lose weight as well as generally improve their quality of life. Unfortunately, many people with a chronic pain condition mistakenly believe they can no longer achieve the full benefits of exercise.

Type, Frequency, and Style

Exercise can and should be part of your pain management plan. The type and frequency of exercise is the important factor, which requires someone with experience and clinical skills to help you develop an effective—and safe—program. Rest and immobilization periods (or up-time and down-time), should also be an integral foundation of your plan.

Other important considerations include the style of exercise, the progression of intensity, the frequency or quantity, and the prevention of additional injury. As mentioned earlier, hydrotherapy and water exercises can be very beneficial for people with chronic pain issues.

Most treatment providers working with pain management believe that mobilization through exercise is an important component of a successful treatment plan. Motion is the way to obtain quick and lasting relief of pain. Exercise helps increase range of motion, which is essential for increasing your mobility and healing.

As mentioned earlier, the development of an exercise program should be done under the direction of a specialist. For some of you this will be your doctor, chiropractor, physical therapist, and/or a personal trainer. Whichever specialist is chosen should become a part of your APM treatment team. Effective communication should be ongoing due to the many exercise difficulties that frequently occur.

Using an exercise specialist is important due to the many different types of pain issues involved, as well as the many different types of exercise modalities available.

Three Types of Exercise
- Isotonic
- Isometric
- Isokinetic

There are basically three types of exercise and each type achieves different results. The first type—**isotonic**—is active muscle contraction, moving a joint partially or thoroughly through its range of motion. Some examples of isotonic exercise include flexing and extending various limbs, with or without using resistance. This can be carried out with either free weights (dumbbells or barbells) or fixed equipment. In both forms exercises are carried out against a fixed resistance. As each muscle moves through its complete range, isotonic contraction creates tension with maximum effort at the beginning and end of each exercise.

The second type is also an active exercise—**isometric**—where the joint remains still during the muscle contraction. Isometric exercise, as it pertains to muscle training, involves tensing muscles against other muscles or against an immovable object while the length of the muscles remains unchanged. Effective isometric training is achieved when the muscle tension is maintained over a certain period of time.

The third type—**isokinetic**—is where resistance is applied to force muscles to exert maximum force throughout the range of motion. Isokinetic exercise is performed with a specialized apparatus that provides variable resistance to a movement so that no matter how much effort is exerted, the movement takes place at a constant speed. Such exercise is used to test and improve muscular strength and endurance, especially after injury. Isokinetic exercise requires specialized equipment.

It's important to practice aerobic exercise at least three times a week to improve health and weight management. Many people with pain fear that their pain will increase if they become too active. However, the risks of not exercising far outweigh the discomfort of developing an appropriate exercise regime. If you are careful and progress slowly, you are not likely to worsen your condition.

Some of the forms of recommended exercise include the following:
- Water exercise
- Stationary bike
- Treadmills

- Walking
- Yoga or Tai Chi
- Indoor cross-country ski equipment

When completely removing your pain is not possible, using exercise can increase your level of functioning, thus improving your quality of life and enabling you to more effectively manage your pain. Another benefit of exercise is the increased ability of your body to produce additional endorphins. As I discussed earlier, these neurotransmitters help your body manage pain.

People who gradually incorporate exercise into their pain-management treatment plan return to a higher functioning level and maintain more effective pain management. An exercise program should also include proper posture and stretching. There is also a secondary gain for exercise—reducing isolation tendencies.

Use Exercise to Socialize

As I mentioned in an earlier chapter, isolation tendencies are common for people with chronic pain. Such was the case for both Donna and Matt. Donna used her hydrotherapy and water exercise classes as a place to socialize and share with people in a similar situation. Matt tended to socialize much less than Donna, but he was able to form a few close relationships with people who frequented the health club he joined.

Exercise and Stress Reduction

Reducing and managing stress is an additional reason for exercise. As I discussed earlier, both Donna and Matt noticed a high correlation between stress and the intensity of their pain symptoms. Each of these patients used their exercise program as an integral part of their stress-management strategy.

Matt noticed that if his stress levels were above a level seven and he would just go swim a few laps, he could then bring his stress level down to a four or five and be able to manage it more effectively. He also noticed that the distress of his pain symptoms decreased at the same time.

In addition to effective stress management, Donna used exercise to help reduce her weight and increase her energy level. She noticed that when she gained weight, her pain symptoms increased. When she followed a proper diet and exercise program, her pain symptoms decreased.

Exercise and Depression

As I discussed earlier, depression is common for people who experience a chronic pain condition. Managing depression is another important reason for a person with chronic pain to exercise.

Many therapists who work with various depressive mood disorders note that a regular exercise program is an important component of the treatment plan, but acknowledge that additional measures may also be needed. These measures could include nutritional changes and even antidepressant medications in some appropriate cases.

Diet and Exercise for Healthy Recovery

In addition to being an important part of an effective pain-management program, a proper nutrition and exercise plan is an essential component of a chemical-dependency recovery plan. When you use psychoactive chemicals for a prolonged period of time biochemical changes occur. Some of those changes were discussed earlier.

When you stop using drugs—whether it's prescription medication, alcohol, or other drugs—you often experience withdrawal symptoms. Fortunately, those symptoms are fairly short lived, from between three days to five or six weeks. Unfortunately, what follows is a period of protracted or post acute withdrawal (PAW). PAW usually lasts between eighteen months to three years. The symptoms of PAW will be discussed in the next chapter.

Effective management for PAW includes a healthy, nutritious diet and regular exercise. When people have an effective pain-management and recovery program in place, their risk of relapse decreases significantly. A proper nutritional and exercise plan needs to be a part of your APM recovery plan, which is further covered in the following chapter.

> **Nutrition and exercise are essential components of relapse prevention.**

An ongoing practice of healthy nutrition and exercise can be difficult to accomplish. Over a prolonged period of time your motivation may diminish, being replaced with boredom, forgetfulness, and distractions. However, an effective relapse prevention plan that includes nutrition and exercise along with the other components covered in the following chapter, will significantly decrease tendencies toward self-sabotage.

Earlier I discussed the importance of using a multidimensional treatment plan because the addiction pain syndrome produces a synergistic effect. This chapter has emphasized the importance of combining the holistic treatment processes and the medication management components. The next chapter covers the importance of using a relapse prevention strategy designed to treat the synergistic effects of the addiction pain syndrome. This process is called **Reciprocal Relapse Prevention**. You will also learn how Donna and Matt completed APM Core Clinical Processes Five and Six.

Chapter Eight

Reciprocal Relapse Prevention

The CENAPS® Model of Relapse Prevention

Chronic pain is a serious problem for many recovering people and often leads to relapse, so relapse prevention planning is crucial in order for you to have a successful treatment outcome.

Over the past decade, relapse prevention planning has become an important component in a number of chemical dependency treatment programs. Many now use the CENAPS® Model of Relapse Prevention developed by Terence T. Gorski—an innovative and dynamic process. This method includes identifying high-risk situations for relapse, training in analysis and management of high-risk situations, developing a relapse prevention network, and constructing an early intervention plan to be implemented if serious signs of relapse appear.

Unfortunately, a literature review did not reveal any medical model pain clinics incorporating intensive relapse prevention plans into their treatment programs. However, other innovative pain programs that use a biopsychosocial approach do include some relapse prevention. The APM System includes an effective relapse prevention component.

> Relapse prevention planning is a crucial component of the APM treatment plan!

This chapter illustrates and explains the APM relapse prevention protocols used by Donna and Matt. This chapter also reviews the relapse prevention exercises from the *Addiction-Free Pain Management Workbook* and shows how Donna and Matt completed that portion of their relapse prevention and recovery planning work.

Redefining Relapse

Progressive Nature of Relapse: From Stability to Dysfunction

Relapse education must start with a new definition of relapse:

> Relapse is a progressive series of events that takes you from stable recovery to a state of becoming dysfunctional in your recovery.

When you start on the slide to relapse you undergo many changes. The first change occurs in your thinking. Recovery-prone positive thinking is replaced by relapse-prone negative thinking and euphoric recall. Euphoric recall is remembering only the payoffs for taking the pain medication while your negative self-talk may say something like, "It's not fair. I can't use it now." The pain and problems you may have experienced are forgotten or repressed.

This negative thinking leads to you experiencing uncomfortable and/or painful emotions. These feelings produce self-defeating urges, which are often followed by self-destructive behaviors. Inappropriate use of pain medication may not be an option in the early stages of relapse, but the negative self-destructive behaviors often set you up to experience more problems and an eventual return to inappropriately using your pain medication in order to cope.

Relapse and Post Acute Withdrawal

One of the biggest relapse triggers in early recovery is your inability to recognize and/or cope with the serious symptoms of protracted or post-acute withdrawal (PAW). PAW is a series of biological and psychological symptoms that everyone in chemical dependency recovery goes through. The brain chemistry is adapting and healing from the long-term toxic effects of psychoactive substance use. In chapter one I explained this toxic effect as *substance-induced organic mental disorders.*

Six Major PAW Symptoms
- Thinking changes
- Emotional changes
- Sleep disturbances
- Short-term and long-term memory problems
- Physical coordination problems
- An extreme sensivity to stress

The accompanying stress, and distress, of a chronic pain condition often amplify post-acute withdrawal symptoms. As I covered in the previous chapter, you need to develop an effective PAW management plan to lessen the impact of these symptoms on your pain management and recovery process.

Relapse Prevention Planning

Relapse prevention starts with assessment and treatment planning followed by a high-risk situation identification process. High-risk situations for people with chronic pain are events that lead to you wanting to use inappropriate pain medication or other drugs (including alcohol) after making a commitment not to relapse. They also include situations that make you want to stop using an effective pain management program despite your promises to yourself to lead a healthy recovery-prone lifestyle.

Identifying and Managing Core Issues

Besides core addiction issues and core psychological issues, you also have to contend with core pain issues. Core addictive issues are problems caused by the addiction itself that would not exist if the addiction had not developed. They create emotional pain and dysfunction and require a recovery plan.

Denial is a prime example of a core addictive issue, and in the case of people in chronic pain, denial is often much stronger. A typical APM person might say, "I can't be a real addict because I have pain and a doctor gave me the meds." Both Donna and Matt had similar mistaken beliefs.

Core psychological issues are reoccurring problems caused by unresolved issues from childhood or unresolved adult trauma. They create a deeply entrenched system of irrational beliefs that coexist with the core addictive issues. Some common examples are post-traumatic stress disorder (PTSD) and clinical depression. In fact, a chronic pain condition will often re-trigger PTSD. This is an area where including a trained psychotherapist on your team can have the greatest effectiveness.

The core pain issues are problems caused by the chronic pain condition and your response to that condition. An example of a core pain issue is the cyclical increase (flare-up) of pain due to the stresses of everyday living.

Relapse Justifications

Relapse justifications are patterns of irrational thinking that create an immediate justification for chemical use.

There are five common/basic justifications:

- Euphoric recall ("It worked in the past so it must be OK now")
- Awfulizing recovery ("Recovery is and always will be a terrible struggle")
- Magical thinking ("Medication will fix me—I don't need to do anything else")
- Low tolerance for frustration ("I can't stand feeling so bad about...")
- Low tolerance for pain—emotional or physical ("I can't stand hurting so much")

One of the most common relapse justifications for people with chronic pain is, "I have a legitimate reason to be in pain. Therefore it's OK to do anything to stop my pain." It's critical for you to learn how to identify and talk back to your relapse justifications and how to manage your warning signs or high-risk situations.

Process Seven (TFUAR Analysis) in the *Addiction-Free Pain Management Workbook* is an ideal tool for teaching you to identify and challenge old ways of coping as well as developing recovery-prone action plans. This process will be described later in this chapter.

The Relapse Prevention Network

For effective warning-sign or high-risk situation management, you need to develop a relapse prevention network. An effective relapse prevention network consists of you, a therapist or counselor, family members and/or significant others, other health care professionals, and appropriate Twelve-Step or other support people (such as a Pills Anonymous sponsor).

You need to work with this network to develop a relapse intervention plan. This is one more way for you to take an active role in your recovery process. You share your relapse triggers with your network and inform each member of what to do if any active triggers and/or symptoms of chemical use arise. Identifying early critical warning signs and sharing that knowledge with your relapse prevention network greatly increases the chances of stopping a relapse process before your actual chemical use begins.

Hish-risk situations are any experiences that activate urges to self-medicate despite your best intentions not to relapse.

As I discussed earlier, relapse prevention counseling starts with assessment and treatment planning followed by a high-risk situation identification process. A high-risk situation is any experience that can activate the urge to use inappropriate pain medication (including alcohol) or other drugs in spite of your commitment not to go back. It can also be a situation that makes you want to stop using your effective pain management program despite your promises to yourself.

The following section explains Process Five in the *Addiction-Free Pain Management Workbook*: The High-Risk Situation exercise.

Process Five: Identifying and Personalizing High-Risk Situations

Defining the concept of a high-risk situation can be tricky. Some situations activate self-defeating or addictive urges for some people and not others. The same situation can activate the urges at some times and not others. Process Five is broken down into three separate parts. Part 1 is designed to help you identify a high-risk situation you will be facing in the near future and then personalize it. You do this by completing the following items from the *Addiction-Free Pain Management Workbook.*

Process Five, Part 1: Identifying Immediate High-Risk Situations

1. **Identify an immediate high-risk situatiom:** Think ahead over the next six weeks and identify a situation that could make you want to use inappropriate pain medication (including alcohol) or other drugs despite your commitment not to. Write a short sentence that describes this situation. What is that situation?

2. **How does this situation increase your risk of using pain medication?** Write a sentence or short paragraph that describes how this situation will make you want to use inappropriate pain medication (including alcohol) or other drugs despite your commitment against it.

3. **Write a personal title:** Write a personal title for that situation (a title is a word or short phrase that identifies the situation).

   Personal Title: _____

4. **Write a personal description:** Write a sentence that describes the high-risk situation. Use this format: *I know that I am in a high-risk situation when <I do something> that causes <pain and problems> and I want to use inappropriate pain medication (including alcohol) or other drugs to manage the pain or to solve the problems.* (*Example:* I know that I am in a high-risk situation when <I stop swimming daily> and that causes <my back to start hurting more> so I want to take a pill to make my pain go away.)

5. **Need for pain medication:** How strongly do you believe that you will be able to avoid using inappropriate pain medication (including alcohol) or other drugs in this situation? (Pick a rating between 0 and 10.)

6. **Why do you rate it that way?**

Donna's High-Risk Situation

Donna identified a situation where she had to meet with her son's schoolteacher about a classroom discipline problem. She recognized that this situation was increasing her stress levels, and when her stress levels rose her pain also increased.

The title she chose was "Here we go again." She completed the sentence this way: "I know I'm in a high-risk situation when I stop my stress management when I'm upset, which causes my pain to get worse and I want to take a pill." She believed she had only a 50-percent chance of avoiding using at this point because she couldn't see any other options.

Matt's High-Risk Situation

Matt chose a situation where he was going to confront his fear of intimacy. He was invited to a Twelve-Step program event by one of the women he had wanted to ask out, but never had the nerve. She ended up inviting him to an upcoming dance.

The title he chose was "stark terror." He reported that he was especially afraid that too much dancing would increase his pain. He completed the sentence this way: "I know I'm in a high-risk situation when I tell myself I need to take something before I go so I can perform and not disappoint my date." He believed that he had a 60-percent chance of not using, but he was still very anxious.

Take a few minutes to complete this exercise in your APM workbook.

Part 2 of Process Five in the Addiction-Free Pain Management Workbook asks you to read the high-risk situation developed specifically for the APM population. The list on the next page contains twenty-three items broken down into ten categories.

Process Five, Part 2: Reading the High-Risk Situation List

☐ **1. We only want to stop because we have problems:** We experience a serious problem or crisis related to our pain medication (including alcohol) or other drug use. We feel an inner conflict. One part of us wants to keep taking the medication despite the problem. Another part of us says no and holds us back, because to keep using would cause even more serious problems. We convince ourselves that it would be a good idea to stop taking the medication until the situation calms down, but we feel deprived. Because we don't believe we can continue to cope with life without our pain medication, we leave the door open to change our mind later when things have calmed down.

☐ **2. We don't see the connection:** We are blind to the relationship between our use of pain medication (including alcohol) or other drugs and the problems that we're having. We convince ourselves that we need to use pain medication despite the problems. Nobody has the right to make us stop. We tell ourselves that the real problem isn't our pain medication—it's the pain we have. Sure we've got some serious problems. That's why we're taking the medication—to help us cope with those problems. Besides, a doctor prescribed it for us, so it must be all right.

☐ **3. We deny we're addicted:** We tell ourselves that we're in control of our pain medication use; it doesn't control us. We can stop forever if only the pain would stop for good. We're not taking the medication now and that proves we're in control. Nobody is going to be able to convince us we're some kind of drug addict.

☐ **4. We push away those who threaten our continued pain medication use:** We prove we're not an addict or drug abuser by telling ourselves we have friends and people who care about us, and they don't mind our using the medication at all. There are other people who don't like us the way we are. It's these people, who aren't really our friends, who want us to stop. If they were really our friends, they wouldn't be causing us problems by sticking their noses in where they don't belong. They would realize we deserve to have the medication. If they'd just leave us alone everything would be fine.

☐ **5. We only remember the good times:** We start remembering how good it was to use our pain medication in the past. We make our memories bigger than life by exaggerating the relief we got while minimizing or blocking out the emotional pain and the negative side effects we experienced. We start to convince ourselves that we always felt good and never experienced any pain or problems when we were taking our pain medication the way we wanted.

☐ **6. We "awfulize" being off pain medication:** We start thinking about how hard it is to stay away from pain medication. We convince ourselves that it is awful, terrible, and unbearable to have to live without using our pain medication. Sober living is nothing but pain, problems, and hassles. Without pain medication we can never have a pain-free, good life.

☐ **7. We use magical thinking:** We believe pain medication can magically fix us. We know that pain medication would make us feel good and solve all our problems. We convince ourselves that this time we won't abuse it or lose control. We'll use it responsibly. Besides, it will be just this one time. We'll only use for a short period of time until the pain settles down. Then we'll stop again.

☐ **8. We recycle addictive thinking:** We keep recycling these three thoughts in our head: *Remember how good it was! Look at how awful it is that I can't! Imagine how good it would be if only I could do it again.* By recycling these thoughts we turn the thought (Wouldn't it be nice if I could), into a desire (I want relief), into an urge (I should be able to get relief), and eventually into a craving (I need to stop the pain now; I have no other choice).

☐ **9. We get into problem situations:** We start putting ourselves into situations that create unnecessary stress, pain, and problems.

a. We make our pain worse: Sometimes we have a legitimate pain flair-up and end up doing things that make it worse instead of better. We shoot ourselves in the foot by not using effective pain management and experience the negative consequences. Then we reload the gun and shoot ourselves in the other foot.

b. We overcommit: Sometimes we take on more than we can handle and start missing deadlines and letting other people down. This causes our stress to increase, leading to our pain going up. Instead of talking openly about the problem, we go underground, put things off, blame others, and try to cover our tracks. If we get caught, we get defensive and try to rationalize our way out of it.

c. We get frustrated: Sometimes we get frustrated because we want something that we can't have: a totally pain-free life. When this happens we feel deprived because we should be able to have it. We deserve it. We're entitled to it. Others don't have the right to keep us from getting it, even if we need to use pain medication to obtain it.

d. We argue and fight: Sometimes we want to have a good time and forget about our problems, so we visit our friends, other family members, or our parents. We end up getting into arguments, fights, or conflicts. We leave believing that no one really cares about us or understands us, which causes our stress and pain to increase.

e. We want to fit in: We feel left out. It seems like no one likes us or wants to be around us when our pain condition limits us. We want to fit in and feel like a normal person, but somehow we just can't see ourselves doing it without using pain medication.

☐ **10. We seek out a pain-medication supportive environment:** We start putting ourselves in situations where we're around people, places, and things that make us want to use pain medication despite our commitment not to.

a. We want to feel better: We might get into situations where we're feeling good but we want to feel even better or enjoy ourselves more. We don't know how without medication.

b. We want to change our energy: We might get into situations that stress us out or make us feel tired and bored. These situations leave us feeling like we need something either to calm us down or pick us up.

c. We hang out with old friends: We might accidentally run into someone who supported our use of pain medication. We might get invited out by friends or family members and feel we can't say no. We don't want to use pain medication, but we can't see ourselves spending time with them without taking something.

d. We see people enjoying themselves: We might be in a social situation. The people we're with are having a very good time and being very active. We suddenly notice that everyone else is doing things that we can't do without taking pain medication. We don't want to use pain medication, but everyone else is having so much fun that we feel pressured. We remember how good it could be and ask ourselves, Why not? Besides, no one will know.

e. We want better sex: We might get into a sexual experience that could be enhanced by using pain medication. Or a sexual experience might not be going as well as we would like. We know that pain medication could improve our performance, increase our pleasure, get rid of our limitations, and help us to seduce or please our partner.

f. We face a loss: A family member or friend might die. We have to go to the funeral and attend the social functions that surround it. We see people using alcohol or other drugs to cope with their pain. One relative is walking around offering tranquilizers to anyone who wants them. We remember that our pain medication could help us feel better, too. Then we go home, alone, to deal with the pain and loss. We want to feel better, but we don't know what to do.

g. We remember the "good old days": We find ourselves daydreaming about how healthy and active we used to be, or sometimes we wake up from dreaming about participating in our old favorite physical activities. When we realize it is only a dream we feel cheated and frustrated. We need to grieve the loss of our healthy self, but we don't know how.

h. We feel trapped: We might get backed into a corner and start feeling trapped because we don't know what to do. We might get into a situation where we feel isolated or cut off from others. It seems there is no way to fit in or get connected. To avoid situations like this, we might start spending more time alone, and when we're by ourselves we might start to feel lonely. When our pain is bad we don't reach out; we suffer all alone.

i. We get sick: We might get sick, injured, or start having different physical pain or discomfort. A doctor might offer us a prescription for pain medication, muscle relaxants, or tranquilizers. What's wrong with that? He's a doctor, we're sick or in pain, and it is different from our other condition. We deserve relief. We don't mention our past problems with pain medication.

This high-risk situation list is an adaptation of the high-risk situation list developed by Terence T. Gorski with the help of Roland Williams, Arthur B. Trundy, Tim Dworniczek, and Joseph E. Troiani. The high-risk situation list is based, in part, on the research of G. Alan Marlatt and Helen Annis.

Take a few minutes to complete this exercise in your APM workbook.

The next exercise in the *Addiction-Free Pain Management Workbook* asks you to use what you learned by reading the high-risk situation list to modify the high-risk situation you chose in Part 1. See the exercise below.

Process Five, Part 3: Discussion Questions

1. What is the high-risk situation you will be facing in the immediate future that could cause you to use inappropriate pain medication (including alcohol) or other drugs despite your commitment not to? (Use the high-risk situation from *Process Five, Part 1: Question 1: Identifying High-Risk Situations.*)

2. What did you learn from reading the APM/RPC High-Risk Situation List that can help you to understand and clarify this high-risk situation?

3. Revise your *personal title* for the high-risk situation. Try to find words that are more descriptive and easier for you to remember. The title should also stir up a feeling or emotion. The title should not be any longer than two or three words. What is your revised personal title for this high-risk situation?

Personal Title: _____

4. Revise your *personal description* for the high-risk situation that you selected. The revised description should still start with the words "I know that I'm in a high-risk situation when...." You should use something you learned by reading the high-risk situation list to make the revised description more concrete and specific. Remember to use the same general format.

Donna's Magical Thinking

Donna identified with the magical thinking high-risk situation number 7: **We use magical thinking:** We believe that pain medication can magically fix us. We know that pain medication would make us feel good and solve all of our problems. We convince ourselves that this time we won't abuse it or lose control. We'll use it responsibly. Besides, it will just be this one time. We'll only use for a short period of time until the pain settles down. Then we'll stop again.

She realized she was using the added stress as an excuse to use pain medication to help her deal with an uncomfortable situation—the way she used to do it. She changed her title to

"Doing it again." She completed the sentence this way: "I know I'm in a high-risk situation when I begin to sabotage my self-care and start remembering how well pills used to help me escape when I'm really upset."

Matt's Wanting Better Sex

Matt chose the situation pertaining to sex (number 10–e): **We want better sex:** We might get into a sexual experience that could be enhanced by using pain medication. Or a sexual experience might not be going as well as we would like. We know that pain medication could improve our performance, increase our pleasure, get rid of our limitations, and help us to seduce or please our partner.

He realized that the dancing was not the issue at all. He was afraid this date would lead to a sexual encounter sometime later and he would embarrass himself by not being able to perform.

He changed his title to "performance anxiety." He revised the sentence this way: "I know I'm in a high-risk situation when I tell myself I can't go on a date unless I take something so I won't embarrass myself in case I get a chance for sex." Matt's sexual dysfunction issue was serious, but now was not the time to attempt resolution, so the process of "Bookmarking" was used.

Using the Bookmarking Technique

Bookmarking is a skill that allows you to identify and clarify secondary issues and problems as they emerge, explore the relationship of those issues to your current target problem, write it down, and agree to work on it later in recovery. Working on his sexual issue too soon could lead Matt to relapse. It was in Matt's best interest to avoid sexual situations at this point in his sobriety.

Using Process Six, *Situation Mapping,* was an appropriate intervention for Matt to deal with the immediate high-risk situation in a safe way. Matt also talked with his sponsor about not being in relationship until he was stable in his recovery.

Process Six: Situation Mapping

Process Six is divided into three parts. Part 1 asks you to think of a specific time when you experienced your high-risk situation and managed it in a way that caused you to use inappropriate pain medication or other drugs (including alcohol) and/or used ineffective pain management. You are asked to tell the experience as if it were a story with a beginning, middle, and end.

Part 2 asks you to think of a specific time when you experienced this high-risk situation and managed it using effective pain management and/or avoided using inappropriate pain medication or other drugs (including alcohol).

In Part 3 you are asked to think of the most important high-risk situation you will be experiencing in the near future. You are asked to imagine yourself using ineffective pain management that will cause you to use inappropriate pain medication or other drugs (including alcohol). Then you are asked to imagine yourself doing the things that you would have done in the past to convince yourself that it's justifiable to use inappropriate pain medication or other drugs (including alcohol).

Both Donna and Matt were able to identify appropriate mapping situations that led them to much more clarity about their past using incidents. By answering the remaining questions in the mapping processes, both Donna and Matt were able to identify three intervention points where they could have done something different to change the outcome. Below are the remainder of the questions for the mapping processes.

Process Six, Parts 1, 2, & 3: Discussion Questions

1. What did you want to accomplish by managing this situation the way you did?

2. Did you get what you wanted by managing the situation in this way?

☐ Yes   ☐ No   ☐ Unsure

Explain:

_____

3. On a scale of 1 to 10, **what were your stress levels** when you managed the situation this way. _____

4. Doing something different: Can you think of some things that you could do differently to manage the situation without having to use inappropriate pain medication (including alcohol) or other drugs?

5. Avoiding the situation: What could you have done to responsibly avoid getting into this situation?

   If you avoided this situation, how would it have changed the outcome?

6. Intervention point #1: What could you have done differently near the beginning of the situation to produce a better outcome? (How could you have thought differently? managed your feelings and emotions differently? fought your self-destructive urges differently? acted or behaved differently? treated other people differently?)

   If you do these things, how will it change the outcome?

7. Intervention point #2: What can you do differently near the middle of the situation to produce a better outcome? (How could you have thought differently? managed your feelings and emotions differently? fought your self-destructive urges differently? Acted or behaved differently? Treated other people differently?)

   If you do these things, how will it change the outcome?

8. Intervention point #3: What can you do differently near the end of the situation to produce a better outcome? (How could you have thought differently? managed your feelings and emotions differently? fought your self-destructive urges differently? acted or behaved differently? treated other people differently?)

   If you do these things, how will it change the outcome?

9. Stop relapse quickly: If you start using inappropriate pain medication (including alcohol) or other drugs, what can you do to stop?

10. Most important thing learned: What is the most important thing that you learned by completing this exercise?

    Note: If you do relapse, it is important not to despair. You can choose to learn from that situation and find that in the future you can intervene before you use inappropriately or experience life-damaging consequences. The important thing is that you learn to intervene as soon as you are able. For some people the recovery process seems to move steadily forward, but for many it goes forward, the person hits a stuck point, consolidates his or her resources, and then moves forward again. Whatever your recovery pattern is, you must not give up. Remember, recovery is a lifelong learning process.

Take a few minutes to complete these exercises in your APM workbook.

Up to now most of this work has been to help you uncover and understand the problems associated with the Addiction Pain Syndrome. In the next chapter you'll see how Donna and Matt learned to further understand and manage their high-risk situations. This is accomplished through the use of the TFUAR Process.

Chapter Nine

Recovery Planning Action Steps

Proooo Seven: Analyzing and Managing High-Risk Situations

TFUAR Analysis

Process Seven in the *Addiction-Free Pain Management Workbook* is TFUAR analysis. As I mentioned earlier, TFUAR stands for thinking, feelings, urges, actions, and reactions (or relationships).

In this exercise you learn how to analyze your high-risk situation by identifying your irrational thoughts, uncomfortable feelings, self-defeating urges, self-destructive actions, and the problematic reactions of others that are related to managing your high-risk situation in a way that could lead you to relapse.

- Thoughts cause feelings
- Thoughts and feelings cause urges
- Urges plus decisions cause actions
- Actions cause reactions from others

Some of you may have difficulty separating your TFUARs. You might not be able to distinguish thoughts from feelings. You may tend to believe that you can think anything you want and it won't affect your feelings. You may not be able to distinguish feelings from urges. You may believe that each feeling carries with it a specific urge. You may not realize that you can experience a feeling, sit still and breathe into the feeling, and that it can dissipate without being acted out. You may not be able to distinguish urges from actions.

Impulse control lives in the space between the urge and the action. This space needs to be expanded (*you can learn to pause and notice the urge but do nothing*), and then filled with **reflection** so that you can begin to question yourself (*What do I have an urge to do? What has happened when I have done similar things in the past? What is likely to happen if I do that now?*) and make an appropriate **decision** (*What do I choose to do? I know I'll be responsible for the action and its consequences*).

Some of you may not be able to distinguish action from social reaction. You may tend to believe that people respond to you for no reason at all. You may not link the responses of others to the behaviors you use with others.

With the above information in mind, let's look at Process Seven in the *Addiction-Free Pain Management Workbook*, which has five parts. Part 1 asks you to list the high-risk situation you're working on and then analyze your TFUARs. The workbook exercises are reproduced below.

Process Seven, Part 1: TFUAR Analysis

1. What is the immediate high-risk situation you are learning to manage?

2. When you are in this high-risk situation, what do you tend to think?

3. Review the list of Addictive Thinking Errors in Process Seven, Part 2. In the first column list three of those thoughts you tend to use in this situation. In the second column below think of another thought you could use to manage this situation without using pain medication (including alcohol) or other drugs.

Addictive thoughts	Sober and responsible thoughts
Thoughts that make me want to use pain medication (including alcohol) or other drugs to cope with the situation.	Thoughts that challenge my addictive way of thinking and encourage me to manage the situation in an effective and healthy way.

---

(1)	(1)
(2)	(2)
(3)	(3)

4. When you are in this high-risk situation, what do you tend to feel?

5. Review the feeling checklist (Process Seven, Part 3). Identify the three primary feelings you tend to have in this high-risk situation: Answer the question beneath each feeling. Read the feeling management skills (Process Seven, Part 4) before identifying new ways of thinking and acting that could help you to manage the feeling more effectively.

Feeling #1:	**Strength of feeling (0–10):**
What I am *thinking* that makes me feel that way is:	Another way of *thinking* that could make me feel different is:
What I am *doing* that makes me feel that way is:	Another way of *acting* that could make me feel different is:
Feeling #2:	**Strength of feeling (0–10):**
What I am *thinking* that makes me feel that way is:	Another way of *thinking* that could make me feel different is:
What I am *doing* that makes me feel that way is:	Another way of *acting* that could make me feel different is:

Feeling #3:	Strength of feeling (0–10):
What I am *thinking* that makes me feel that way is:	Another way of *thinking* that could make me feel different is:
What I am *doing* that makes me feel that way is:	Another way of *acting* that could make me feel different is:

6. When you are in this high-risk situation, what do you have an urge to do?

   A. Is there one part of you that wants to use inappropriate pain medication (including alcohol) or other drugs? Please describe that part of you.

   B. Is there one part of you that wants to manage the situation without using pain medication (including alcohol) or other drugs? Please describe that part of you.

   C. If you wanted to solve the problem you are currently facing, which part of you do you need to listen to and why?

7. When you experience this high-risk situation, what do you actually do?

8. Review the list of Addictive Behaviors (Process Seven, Part 5) and list the three primary addictive behaviors you tend to use to cope with this situation and something that you could do instead that would produce a better outcome.

Addictive behaviors	Sober and responsible behaviors
Things I do that stop me from learning how to deal with life without using inappropriate pain medication (including alcohol) and other drugs.	Things I do that help me manage feelings and situations using appropriate and healthy pain management responses.
(1)	(1)
(2)	(2)

(3)	(3)

9. When you used the addictive behaviors listed, how did other people react?

   A. Can you think of some of the ways people reacted to you that increased your risk of using inappropriate pain medication (including alcohol) and other drugs?

   B. Can you think of some of the ways that people reacted to you that helped you to choose more appropriate pain management alternatives or find healthier options?

10. Most important thing learned: What is the most important thing you learned by completing this exercise?

Donna and Matt experienced some confusion working on the above exercise but were able to eventually work through their stuck points. It's important for you to work with a professional who has been trained in the CENAPS® model to get the greatest benefits from these workbook exercises. If that isn't possible any therapist or counselor with chemical dependency experience can also be helpful. The important thing is to share this work with a trusted person who can give you constructive feedback.

TFUAR Management

Part 1 of this exercise asks you to refer ahead to the exercises in Parts 2 through 5, which are listed below. Think of these processes as tools. These tools are designed to help you better understand and complete the exercises in Part 1.

Part 2 asks you to think of the high-risk situation that you want to learn how to manage without using inappropriate pain medication and/or other drugs (including alcohol). You are asked to read each of the addictive thoughts listed below and ask yourselves if you tend to think similar thoughts when you are in the high-risk situation. If you do, check the box in front of the thought(s) you picked. It's also helpful to rate each addictive thought on a scale of 0 to 10 with 0 meaning you never have this type of thinking to 10 meaning this type thinking is very common for you.

Process Seven, Part 2: Identifying Addictive Thoughts

☐ 1. I have a right to use any medication I want and nobody has the right to tell me to stop.

☐ 2. I don't have problems because of pain medication. I use pain medication to cope with problems.

☐ 3. I have pain medication problems, but they're not that bad.

☐ 4. I have pain medication problems, but I have a good reason for having them!

☐ 5. I have pain medication problems, but it's not my fault!

☐ 6. I always feel good and never feel bad or have problems when I'm using pain medication.

☐ 7. I always feel bad and have a lot of pain and problems when I'm not using pain medication.

☐ 8. Pain medication can magically fix me and solve my problems.

☐ 9. Pain medication is good for me and lets me feel good and have a better quality of life.

☐ 10. Not using pain medication is bad for me, makes me feel bad, and stops me from having a good life.

☐ 11. Pain medication always makes me feel good. It never makes me feel bad.

☐ 12. Not using pain medication always makes me feel bad. It never makes me feel good.

☐ 13. Pain medication lets me do things I can't do without it.

☐ 14. Not using pain medication stops me from doing things I could do if I were using pain medication.

☐ 15. Pain medication lets me handle pain and solve problems I couldn't manage without it.

☐ 16. Not using pain medication causes me increased pain and problems I wouldn't have if I were using pain medication.

17. Pain medication makes it easy for me to deal with people and build relationships.

18. Not using pain medication makes it hard for me to deal with people and build relationships.

19. I am in control of my pain medication use. It does not control me.

20. I can stop any time I want to. I just don't want to because there's really no good reason to stop.

21. I must control my pain medication use or I will be no good.

22. People who support my use of pain medication are my friends.

23. People who criticize my use of pain medication are my enemies.

Donna's Addictive Thoughts Selections

On this exercise Donna picked numbers 1, 5, 8, 9, 13, 15, 17, 18, and 21. This exercise helped her to see a previously unconscious process that led to the inappropriate use of her pain medication. She especially focused on items 15, 17, and 18, because relationship issues have always been very difficult for her.

Matt's Addictive Thoughts Selections

Matt chose the following items: 2, 3, 5, 6, 7, 8, 9, 13, 14, 15, 17, 18, 19, 21, and 23. Matt was very surprised at how many of these thoughts he experiences when he is in high-risk situations. His special focus items were 2, 13, and 21, with 21 being the one that produced the most discomfort for him.

Part 3 is the same feeling checklist that was previously covered in an earlier chapter. This time both Donna and Matt saw some differences.

The feelings Donna and Matt chose in the Process One, Part 3 exercise were: weak, angry, sad, lonely, threatened, and frustrated. Donna rated weak at level 10 while Matt rated it level 5. Donna rated sad at level 8 and Matt rated it at 4. Both rated anger and frustration at a level 10, and Donna rated ashamed at level 10 while Matt did not rate either proud or ashamed. This time

Matt was able to see that ashamed was near level 10, and his sad rating moved up to level 8. Both rated lonely at level 10 this time.

Process Seven, Part 3: Feeling Checklist

When you are in this high-risk situation do you tend to feel...

☐ Strong   or   ☐ Weak? How strong is the feeling? (0–10) _____

Why do you rate it that way?

_____

When you are in this high-risk situation do you tend to feel...

☐ Caring   or   ☐ Angry? How strong is the feeling? (0–10) _____

Why do you rate it that way?

_____

When you are in this high-risk situation do you tend to feel...

☐ Happy   or   ☐ Sad?   How strong is the feeling? (0–10) _____

Why do you rate it that way?

_____

When you are in this high-risk situation do you tend to feel...

☐ Safe   or   ☐ Threatened?   How strong is the feeling? (0–10)

_____

Why do you rate it that way?

_____

When you are in this high-risk situation do you tend to feel...

☐ Fulfilled or   ☐ Frustrated?   How strong is the feeling? (0–10)

_____

Why do you rate it that way?

_____

When you are in this high-risk situation do you tend to feel...

☐ Connected   or   ☐ Lonely?   How strong is the feeling? (0–10)

_____

Why do you rate it that way?

_____

When you are in this high-risk situation do you tend to feel...

☐ Proud   or   ☐ Ashamed?   How strong is the feeling? (0–10)

                                                    _____

Why do you rate it that way?

_____

Both Donna and Matt were very happy to see Part 4, The Feeling Management Skills, listed below. Through this exercise they began to see they could learn to manage their feelings.

The instructions for this exercise require you to read each statement and rate how true it is for you on a scale of 0–10; 0 means the statement is not at all true for you, and 10 means the statement is totally true for you.

Process Seven, Part 4: Feeling Management Skills

_____ 1.   I am able to anticipate situations that are likely to provoke strong feelings and emotions.

_____ 2.   I am able to recognize when I am starting to have a strong feeling or emotion.

_____ 3.   I am able to stop myself from automatically reacting to the feeling without thinking it through.

_____ 4.   I am able to call a time-out in emotionally charged situations before my feelings become unmanageable.

_____ 5.   I am able to use an immediate relaxation technique to bring down the intensity of the feeling.

_____ 6.   I am able to take a deep breath and notice what I'm feeling.

_____ 7.   I am able to find words that describe what I'm feeling and use the feeling checklist when necessary.

_____ 8.   I am able to rate the intensity of my feelings using a ten-point scale.

_____ 9. I am able to consciously acknowledge the feeling and its intensity by saying to myself, "Right now I'm feeling _____and it's okay to be feeling this way."

_____ 10. I am able to identify what I'm thinking that's making me feel this way. I ask myself, "How can I change my thinking in a way that will make me feel better?"

_____ 11. I am able to identify what I'm doing that's making me feel this way. I ask myself, "How can I change what I'm doing in a way that will make me feel better?"

_____ 12. I am able to recognize and resist urges to create problems, hurt myself, or hurt other people.

_____ 13. I am able to recognize my resistance to doing things that would help me or my situation, and I force myself to do those things despite the resistance.

_____ 14. I am able to get outside myself and recognize and respond to what other people are feeling.

_____ 15. I am able to seek help when I need help dealing with my feelings.

_____ 16. I am able to talk to significant others or helpers about my feelings.

_____ 17. I am able to express my feelings directly and specifically.

_____ 18. I am able to express my feelings in a way that does not harm myself or others.

Learning Feeling Management Skills

Donna noted that before she started APM treatment she would not have been able to have any items near level 10, but now she had three at level 10: items 1, 5, and 8.

Matt had a similar reaction to this exercise. In the past he tended to be a victim of his feelings and would often use pain medication to cope with his uncomfortable emotions. The three most important management skills for him were items 3, 12, and 15. Number 15, seeking help to deal with feelings, was a major step forward in Matt's recovery.

The final exercise in Process Seven concerns identifying addictive tactics that you have used in the past. In this exercise you are asked to read a list of resistant behavioral tactics that you can use to creatively avoid doing the things you know you need to do in order to recover. You're asked to check the tactic(s) that you have used in the past. Again, it's also helpful to rate each addictive behavior on a scale of 0 to 10 with 0 meaning you never use this type of tactic to 10 meaning this type of behavior is very common for you.

Process Seven, Part 5: Addictive Behaviors

I agree that I need to do something, and then...

☐ 1. I play "Yes, But" by procrastinating, finding excuses to keep putting it off, or finding reasons why I shouldn't have to do it.

☐ 2. I get "Too Busy" to do it.

☐ 3. I play "I'll Wait Until" by expecting something else to happen before I can do what I need to do.

☐ 4. I say "It's Not That Important" and convince myself of all the reasons why other things are more important.

☐ 5. I pretend "I'm Cured" and because I'm OK now I don't need to do what I agreed to do. I agree to keep it in mind if I ever need it.

☐ 6. I play "Trivial Pursuit" by getting sidetracked into doing other low-priority tasks and busywork so that I don't have time to do what I need to do.

☐ 7. I rescue others by finding someone in trouble and play "Rescuer" by shifting the focus from my own recovery to saving them.

☐ 8. I play "Persecution" by finding someone I don't like and criticizing, attacking, and blaming them for not letting me do what I need to do.

☐ 9. I play "Dumb" and get confused about what I'm supposed to do. No matter how clearly it's explained I just can't understand.

☐ 10. I get overwhelmed, feel scared, and start to feel panic. I use my fear as an excuse not to do what I need to do.

☐ 11. I play "Helpless" by pretending to be too weak and powerless to do what I agreed to do.

☐ 12. I set myself up to be victimized by playing "Poor Me," asking untrustworthy people for help. When no one rescues me I use it as an excuse for not doing what I need to do.

☐ 13. I demand a guaranteed "Quick Fix" or nothing. If it won't instantly fix the problem, I won't even try it.

This exercise is an effective tool for helping you uncover previously unconscious scripts that you have played out over and over again in the past. The first step toward change is recognition that a problem exists. If you are familiar with Transactional Analysis (TA) you may recognize some of the above tactics. Some of the TA tools can be extremely effective in enhancing your recovery process, and many therapists are familiar with those tools.

> ## Donna and Matt learned to identify and overcome self-defeating behavior.

When Donna and Matt saw some of the tactics they have used in front of them on the paper, they started to realize how self-destructive those behaviors were to their recovery process. Donna's most significant realization was seeing a pattern she played out when getting to item 12—"poor me." She was able to look at several of her past significant relationships and saw how she would pick untrustworthy people to ask for help—then she could justify using when they let her down.

> ## Treatment works best when you become more proactive in your healing.

Matt's most important awareness was item 13—the "quick fix" or instant gratification. He was able to identify times in the past that if he had stuck to his pain management plan he would have been able to avoid using—but he stated, "I wanted it now." The process of analyzing and learning to manage high-risk situations is yet another tool to assist you to move from victimization to empowerment.

> Take a few minutes to complete these
> exercises in your APM workbook.

Process Eight: Recovery Planning

Developing a Recovery Plan

The last clinical process in the *Addiction-Free Pain Management Workbook* is focused on recovery planning. Having insight and understanding is only the starting point for successful relapse prevention. Developing an effective recovery plan and following it makes the difference between treatment success or failure for most APM patients.

While the remainder of this chapter explains recovery planning, the next chapter describes measuring treatment effectiveness. Process Eight in the *Addiction-Free Pain Management Workbook* assists you to develop and then test your recovery plan.

Having a structured daily plan assists you in your recovery process and helps you to practice more effective pain management. The recovery activities suggested in Process Eight, Part 1 are a combination of clinical and self-help activities.

These recovery principles are proven by the outcome studies from hundreds of chemical dependency treatment centers across the United States, and by the successful recovery of millions of people working Twelve-Step recovery programs around the world.

> Effective pain management requires a
> recovery pain management plan.

Along the same lines, people who are most effective with their pain management have learned to develop a recovery/ pain management plan. However, it's important to note that this plan needs to be individualized to obtain maximum efficiency. Building a personalized recovery, pain management, and relapse prevention plan is essential for your optimal treatment success. Many times additional motivational counseling is needed to assist you in seeing why all this planning is needed and how it will pay off for you in the end.

Refer to the Addiction Pain Syndrome Diagram, which was first introduced in chapter two. The relapse prevention plan must address all three of the zones in that diagram: the addictive disorder zone, the pain disorder zone, and the addiction pain syndrome zone.

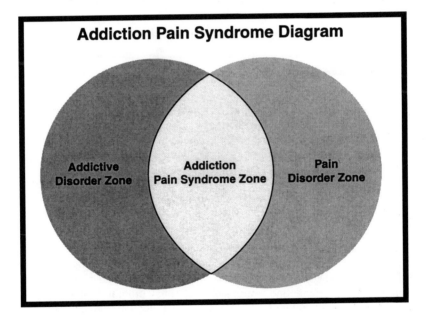

Addiction Pain Syndrome Diagram

Addictive Disorder Zone

Addiction Pain Syndrome Zone

Pain Disorder Zone

There are seven basic recovery activities described below that address these three zones. They are actually habits of good, healthy living. If you want to live a responsible, healthy, and fulfilling life you need to get in the habit of regularly doing these things.

For people in recovery these activities are essential. For those of you who also have a chronic pain disorder (Addiction Pain Syndrome), these steps become even more crucial. A regular schedule of these activities, designed to match your unique profile of recovery needs, pain-management requirements, and high-risk situation management, is necessary for your brain and body to heal from the damage caused by your substance use and your chronic pain condition.

In this exercise you are instructed to read the list of recovery activities below and identify which activities you think will be helpful for your recovery and pain-management program. You are asked to notice the obstacles you may face in practicing them on a regular basis and indicate your strategies to overcome those obstacles. You are then asked if you will put the activities on your recovery plan and why you believe it's important.

The seven recovery activities are listed below.

Process Eight, Part 1: Selecting Recovery Activities

1. Professional Counseling: The success of your recovery and effective pain management will depend on regular attendance at education sessions, group therapy sessions, and individual therapy sessions. The scientific literature on treatment effectiveness clearly shows that the more time you invest in professional counseling and therapy during the first two years of recovery the more likely you are to stay in recovery. This process needs to include pain-management treatment planning.

2. Self-Help Programs: There are a number of self-help programs—such as Alcoholics Anonymous (AA), Pills Anonymous (PA), Chronic Pain Support Groups, Narcotics Anonymous (NA), Rational Recovery, and Women for Sobriety—that can support you in your efforts to live a sober and responsible life. These programs all have several things in common: (1) they ask you to abstain from alcohol and drugs and to live a responsible life; (2) they encourage you to attend meetings regularly so you can meet and develop relationships with other people living sober and responsible lives; (3) they ask you to meet regularly with an established member of the group (usually called a sponsor) who will help you learn about the organization and get through the rough spots; and (4) they promote a program of recovery (often in the form of steps or structured exercises for you to work on outside of meetings) that focuses on techniques for changing your thinking, emotional management, urge management, and behavior.

Scientific research shows that the more committed and actively involved you are in self-help groups during the first two years of recovery, the greater your ability to avoid relapse. You should also consider joining a Chronic Pain Support Group because research indicates that personal empowerment is crucial for developing effective, long-term, chronic-pain management.

3. Proper Diet: What you eat can affect how you think, feel, and act. Many chemically dependent people find they feel better if they eat three well-balanced meals a day, use vitamin and amino acid supplements, avoid eating sugar and foods made with white flour, and cut back or stop smoking cigarettes and drinking beverages containing caffeine, such as coffee and colas. Recovering people who don't follow these simple principles of healthy diet and meal planning tend to feel anxious and depressed, have strong and violent mood swings, feel constantly angry and resentful, and periodically experience powerful cravings. They're more likely to relapse. Those who follow a proper diet tend to feel better and have lower relapse rates. Proper nutrition is also crucial for effective pain management.

4. Exercise Program: If your chronic pain condition permits, doing thirty minutes of aerobic exercise each day will help your brain recover and help you feel better about yourself. Fast walking, jogging, swimming, and aerobics classes are all helpful. It's also helpful to do strength-building exercises (such as weightlifting) and flexibility exercises (such as stretching) in addition to the aerobic exercise. You need to work with your doctor or health-care practitioner to determine the most effective (and safest) exercise program for you.

5. Stress Management Program: Stress is a major cause of relapse. In addition, an increase in stress often leads to an increase in pain. Recovering people who learn how to manage stress without using self-defeating behaviors tend to stay in recovery and learn how to more effectively manage their chronic pain symptoms. Those who don't learn to manage stress tend to relapse or suffer more with their pain. Stress management involves learning relaxation exercises and taking quiet time on a daily basis to relax. It also involves avoiding long hours of working and taking time for recreation and relaxation. Meditation can also be part of this program.

6. Spiritual Development Program: Human beings have both a physical self (based on the health of our brains and bodies) and a nonphysical self (based on the health of our value systems and spiritual lives). Most recovering people find they need to invest regular time in developing themselves spiritually (in other words, exercising the nonphysical aspects of who they are). Twelve-Step programs such as AA provide an excellent program for spiritual recovery as do many communities of faith and spiritual programs. At the heart of any spiritual program are three activities: (1) fellowship, during which you spend time talking with other people who use similar methods; (2) private prayer and meditation, during which you take time alone to be conscious of yourself in the presence of your Higher Power or to consciously reflect on your spiritual self; and (3) group worship, during which you pray and meditate with other people who share a similar spiritual philosophy.

7. Morning and Evening Inventories: People who avoid relapse and successfully obtain lifelong recovery learn how to break free of automatic and unconscious self-defeating responses. They learn to live consciously each day, being aware of what they're doing and taking responsibility for what they do and its consequences. To stay consciously aware, they take time each morning to plan their day (a morning planning inventory), and they take time each evening to review their progress and problems (an evening review inventory). They discuss what they learn about themselves with other people who are involved in their recovery program.

For people with chronic pain, keeping a pain journal identifies stress and trigger patterns as well as associated thoughts, feelings, and behaviors. During times of increased pain, keeping a daily pain journal is essential and leads to more effective pain management.

Take a few minutes to complete this exercise in your APM workbook.

Process Eight, Part 2: The Schedule of Recovery Activities

Once you have identified the recovery activities that are essential to avoid relapse, you need to develop a schedule. Process Eight, Part 2 assists you with that by introducing a weekly planner.

You're given the following instructions:

On the next page is a weekly planner that will allow you to create a schedule of weekly recovery and pain-management activities. Think of a typical week and enter the pain-management and recovery activities that you plan to routinely schedule in the correct time slot for each day. Recovery activities and/or pain-management activities are specific things you do at scheduled times on certain days. If you can't enter the activity onto a daily planner at a specific time, it's not a recovery and/or pain-management activity. Most people find it helpful to have more than one scheduled activity for each day.

Take a few minutes to complete this exercise in your APM workbook.

Once you have developed the calendar, the next step is Part 3, testing the scheduled events. You're asked to complete the exercise listed below.

Process Eight, Part 3:
Testing the Schedule of Recovery Activities

1. Go back to Process 5: Identifying and Personalizing High-Risk Situations and review the primary high-risk situation that you want your recovery and pain-management program to help you identify and manage. Read the personal title and description, and the thought, feeling, urge, and action statements carefully. What is the personal title and description of this high-risk situation?

   Title: _____

   Description: *I know I'm in a high-risk situation when....*

2. Review your CENAPS® Weekly Planner. What is *the most important* recovery and/or pain-management activity that will help you manage this high-risk situation?

   A. How can you use this recovery and/or pain-management activity to help you identify this high-risk situation should it occur? (Remember, most high-risk situations develop in an automatic and unconscious way. A trigger is activated, and we start using the old ways of thinking and acting without being consciously aware of what we're doing. To prevent relapse it's helpful to

179

regularly schedule recovery and/or pain-management activities that will encourage us to talk about how we're thinking, feeling, and acting, and then receive feedback if we experience high-risk situations.)

B. If you start to experience this high-risk situation again, how can you use this recovery activity to manage it? (Remember managing a high-risk situation means changing how you think, feel, and act. How can this recovery activity help you stop thinking and doing things that make you feel like relapsing? How can it help you start thinking and doing things that make you want to get back into recovery?)

3. Review your CENAPS® Weekly Planner again. What is *the second most important* recovery activity that will help you manage this high-risk situation?

A. How can you use this recovery activity to help you to identify this high-risk situation should it occur?

B. If you start to experience this high-risk situation again, how can you use this recovery activity to manage it?

4. Review your CENAPS® Weekly Planner one last time. What is *the third most important* recovery activity that will help you manage this high-risk situation?

A. How can you use this recovery activity to help you identify this high-risk situation should it occur?

B. If you start to experience this high-risk situation again, how can you use this recovery activity to manage it?

5. What other recovery activities can you think of that could be more effective in helping you identify and manage this high-risk situation should it occur?

Take a few minutes to complete this exercise in your APM workbook.

Pain Medication Management Action Plan

Another useful tool for someone in recovery for pain and substance use is a twelve-item protocol for managing pain medication in recovery developed by Stephen F. Grinstead and Sheila Thares. This information (listed below) was introduced to both Donna and Matt who eventually used it very effectively.

Managing Pain Medication in Recovery

For someone recovering from chemical dependency, the use of mood-altering prescription medication can often lead to relapse. The primary goal of this information is for you to learn how to develop a plan that will prevent your sabotaging an effective recovery program, while at the same time avoiding other addiction problems or a destructive pattern of relapse (i.e., ineffective pain management and/or abuse of your pain medication).

This information is a result of many years of study, researching literature on outcome-based treatment, and personal experience. It's designed for people with chronic pain who may need to use psychoactive medication. It is also for people recovering from any chemical dependency who are facing an invasive surgical procedure (medical or dental) that could entail the use of psychoactive medication. It can be helpful to others who may not be in recovery, but have some risk factors for dependency and want to avoid becoming chemically dependent. Included in this information are some strategic action steps that you can take to safely and effectively prepare yourself for an upcoming surgical procedure or other situations requiring the use of psychoactive pain medication.

To accomplish these goals you'll need to do more than just read this twelve-point checklist. You need to discuss your responses to each of the guidelines below with another trusted person who can help you sort out the thoughts and feelings that may surface as a result of these exercises. If you don't have a counselor, you can do this work with the assistance of a self-help group sponsor or trusted significant other who is willing to support you through this process. Discussing what you're learning from this process with another person or a group of people will improve your ability to develop a plan that will prevent relapse.

When you are in recovery for chemical dependency, whether the substance be prescription drugs, alcohol, marijuana, etc., the risk of relapse is always present. One issue that tends to be especially problematic and a relapse trigger for recovering alcoholics and/or addicts is pain. If you have a chronic pain condition, relapse prevention becomes even more crucial. Below are guidelines for people who want to minimize their risk of relapse or inappropriate use of medication.

Personal Action Steps

1. During early recovery postpone non-urgent dental work (except preventative or restorative) and elective surgical procedures requiring mind-altering medications. When you do need to be on medication, make sure that an addiction-medicine practitioner/specialist is used for consultation and/or prescribing that medication.

2. If you need to be on medication, have your sponsor, significant other, or an appropriate support person hold and dispense the medication. Keep only a twenty-four-hour supply available. In the case of a chronic condition requiring ongoing medication, additional precautions must be developed and it's important to use the Recovery and Relapse Indicator Checklist covered earlier.

3. Consult with an addiction-medicine practitioner/specialist about using even non-addictive medications such as an anti-inflammatory, or other over-the-counter analgesics.

4. Be open to exploring all nonpharmacological pain management modalities—the Holistic Components covered earlier. Some of the more common ones are acupuncture, chiropractic, physical therapy, massage therapy, and hydrotherapy. In addition, identifying and managing uncomfortable emotions may also decrease your pain significantly.

5. Be aware of your stress levels and have a stress-management program such as meditation, exercise, relaxation, music, etc. in place. If you lower your stress, you will usually lower your pain as a result.

6. Take personal responsibility to augment your support-group meetings in order to decrease isolation as well as coping with urges and cravings.

7. Inform all of your health-care providers about being in recovery and be aware of the importance of consulting with an addiction-medicine practitioner/specialist in the event that mind-altering medication is needed. There may be times you need to be on medication, but the risk of relapse can be minimized if open communication is maintained between the addiction-medicine practitioner/specialist, yourself, and other health-care providers.

8. Do not overwork, especially if you are in pain or sick. Add one extra day off to your return to work plan to avoid fatigue and promote healing.

9. Be open and aware of the cross-addiction concept. Decline "helpful" offers to use someone else's prescriptions. Any psychoactive chemical could trigger a relapse of your addiction because all mood-altering drugs enter the limbic system as dopamine. This explains why people addicted only to alcohol can relapse back to alcohol after receiving opiates, or an opiate addict can relapse back to opiates after drinking alcohol.

10. Because depression is common for people with chronic pain, consider the possibility of taking appropriate antidepressants if needed.

11. Be aware of the importance of proper nutrition and exercise as a vital part of chronic pain recovery. Stretch slowly at first, then structure progressive walking at least once a day, or twice if necessary to complete the designated distance. Increase the distance as you are able. Add strengthening exercises if cleared by your health-care provider. Remember, protein assists the healing of injuries, therefore it's important to create a nutrition plan for tissue repair.

12. Explore your past beliefs and role models from childhood regarding pain and pain management. Look for healthy role models for pain management in recovery.

You now need to develop your own personal action plan using the above twelve points as a starting place. You need to share your completed plan with your support network and get constructive feedback and modify your plan if needed.

The next chapter covers the measurement of treatment outcomes as well as discussing the last process in the *Addiction-Free Pain Management Workbook,* a final evaluation While Process Nine is not a clinical process per say, it is an important indicator of treatment success or problems.

> An ounce of Relapse Prevention Planning is worth a pound of treatment cure.

The important thing to remember with relapse prevention is the old saying, "An ounce of prevention is worth a pound of cure." You need to understand how important it is not to wait until you are in trouble with your recovery to get active.

It's helpful to look at a relapse prevention plan like a car insurance policy. Many people are fortunate to never have to collect on that insurance, but it sure is nice to know it's available if you have an accident and need it. A solid relapse prevention plan works the same way. You may never need to use the interventions you set up, but should you start that downward spiral toward relapse, it will be comforting to know that you have a plan in place to put on the brakes.

> Relapse prevention is simple, but it's not easy.

Like many other things in recovery, relapse prevention is simple—but not easy. And although relapse prevention is an inside job, that does not mean you have to do it alone. Help is out there for those who need it and want it.

However, you have a much better chance of quality recovery when you use a combination of the APM *core clinical processes,* combined with the as needed *medication management components*, and appropriate *holistic treatment processes*. It's your responsibility to be aware of all potential resources in your communities and seek additional team members when needed.

In the next chapter I discuss how successful treatment is measured. You will learn Donna and Matt's final treatment outcomes. The last process in the *Addiction-Free Pain Management Workbook* is also described in the closing chapter. This exercise is designed to help you complete a final evaluation to learn how much you have benefited from all your work. This is a useful tool to help you see the effectiveness of your treatment process.

Chapter Ten

Measuring Treatment Effectiveness

Determining the effectiveness of chemical dependency treatment is relatively straightforward. If you remain abstinent from alcohol and other psychoactive drugs, the treatment is deemed successful. Determining the outcome of APM treatment is much more complex.

It's not enough for you to achieve abstinence from inappropriate medication. You must also experience an improvement in your pain condition and quality of life. In addition, you must have a solid relapse prevention and pain-management plan that you continue to evaluate and modify frequently.

Benchmarks for Effective Treatment

You need to schedule follow-up reviews with your team to be completed at different intervals, using specific benchmarks that gauge successful treatment. The first follow-up occurs at the completion of the APM process, followed by reviews at three months, six months, nine months, and one year.

These benchmarks include assessing improvement in your quality of life. Improvements are determined by such factors as your returning to work, or other significant increases in the quality of your life as well as the absence, or significant reduction, of psychoactive drug use. Family members and significant others should be asked for their input.

To be considered a total treatment success the following criteria must be met: After one year you must be taking no inappropriate addictive chemicals, report an increase in your quality of life, and report a decrease both in your inactivity due to pain and in your pain levels.

However, it is important to realize that in some cases the most optimal outcome will be a reduction in your medication— or changing to a safer and more effective medication—not total elimination.

Successful APM Treatment Criteria
- Reduction or elimination of addictive medication
- Pain symptoms are decreased
- Quality of Life is increased

You need to learn an effective method to evaluate and rate your progress. Process Nine in the *Addiction-Free Pain Management Workbook* offers such a tool. After completing the first eight clinical processes in the workbook, you then have a chance to complete a final evaluation. Below is the final process that you are instructed to complete.

Process Nine: Final Evaluation

Instructions: The ultimate test of whether you have benefited from completing the exercises in this workbook will be your ability to increase effective pain management and avoid relapse. It may be helpful, however, to review what you have accomplished. A careful evaluation may help you identify areas in your relapse prevention plan that are incomplete. By going back and completing these areas, you may avoid unnecessary relapse and the resulting pain and problems.

Here is a checklist that can help you decide if you have accomplished the objectives of completing this workbook. Read each statement and ask yourself if you have fully completed that objective, partially completed it, or not completed it at all. *Remember:* This is a self-evaluation designed to help you determine if you have the skills needed to avoid relapse. Be honest with yourself. If you relapse because you haven't learned the skills to stay in recovery, you are the one who will pay the price.

1. **The Effects of Chronic Pain:** I understand and can explain the common effects of chronic pain, and the main effects that I personally experienced.

Level of Completion: ☐ None (0)   ☐ Partial (5)   ☐ Full (10)

Score (0–10): ___

2. **The Effects of Prescription and/or Other Drugs** *(including alcohol):* I understand and can explain the benefits I obtained from using prescription or other drugs, and what I wanted to get from using those chemicals. I can also understand and explain the problems I experienced as a result of using.

Level of Completion: ☐ None (0)   ☐ Partial (5)   ☐ Full (10)

Score (0–10): ___

3. **Decision Making about Pain Medication:** I understand and can explain the reasons why I started using pain medication, alcohol, or other drugs. I understand and can explain the reasons why I stopped using pain medication, including alcohol, and other drugs as well as what I did to stay clean and sober.

Level of Completion: ☐ None (0)   ☐ Partial (5)   ☐ Full (10)

Score (0–10): ___

4. **Abstinence Contract and Intervention Planning:** I can define what my abstinence and recovery plan includes. I have completed and signed an abstinence contract, agreeing to maintain abstinence and effective pain management. I have developed an intervention plan that describes the responsibilities of myself, my counselor, and significant others (2 or 3) to stop relapse quickly should it occur.

Level of Completion: ☐ None (0)   ☐ Partial (5)   ☐ Full (10)

Score (0–10): ___

5. **Identifying High-Risk Situations:** I am able to identify the immediate high-risk situations that can cause me to use inappropriate pain medication (including alcohol) or other drugs and/or stop using an effective pain-management program despite my commitment not to, by developing an *Initial High-Risk Situation List* and identifying my immediate high-risk situations.

Level of Completion: ☐ None (0)   ☐ Partial (5)   ☐ Full (10)

Score (0–10): ___

6. **Personalizing High-Risk Situations:** I am able to concretely and specifically describe the immediate high-risk situations, having developed meaningful:

• Personal titles
• Personal descriptions

Level of Completion: ☐ None (0)   ☐ Partial (5)   ☐ Full (10)

Score (0–10): ___

7. **Mapping Past Mismanaged High-Risk Situations:** I am able to use Situation Mapping to objectively describe past high-risk situations that were managed in a way that led to using inappropriate pain medication (including alcohol) or other drugs.

Level of Completion: ☐ None (0)   ☐ Partial (5)   ☐ Full (10)
Score (0–10): ___

8. **Analyzing Past Mismanaged High-Risk Situations:** I am able to use High-Risk Analysis to identify the thoughts, feelings, urges, actions, and relationship patterns caused by the past mismanagement of the high-risk situation.

Level of Completion: ☐ None (0)   ☐ Partial (5)   ☐ Full (10)
Score (0–10): ___

9. **Managing High-Risk Thoughts and Feelings:** I am able to: (1) identify the general way of thinking that is driving situational misman-agement; (2) show the relationship between these thoughts and the feelings driving mismanagement; and (3) use positive self-talk tech-niques to challenge the thoughts and feelings driving situational mismanagement.

Level of Completion: ☐ None (0)   ☐ Partial (5)   ☐ Full (10)
Score (0–10): ___

10. **Mapping Future High-Risk Situations:** I can identify and map future high-risk situations, identify similar past situations that were managed without using alcohol or drugs, identify the critical interven-tion points in those situations, and use new thoughts and behaviors that will allow me to manage the situation by using an appropriate pain-management plan and/or avoid using problematic pain medication (including alcohol) or other drugs.

Level of Completion: ☐ None (0)   ☐ Partial (5)   ☐ Full (10)
Score (0–10): ___

11. **Developing a Recovery Plan:** I am able to develop a schedule of recovery activities that will support my ongoing identification and management of high-risk situations and help me to intervene early should relapse occur.

Level of Completion: ☐ None (0)   ☐ Partial (5)   ☐ Full (10)
Score (0–10): ___

12. **Overall Skill Level:** I have developed an overall ability to identify and manage my high-risk situations that lead me from stable recovery to relapse, and have developed a schedule of recovery activities that will support my ongoing high-risk situation identification and management.

Level of Completion: ☐ None (0)   ☐ Partial (5)   ☐ Full (10)
Score (0–10): ___

If you identified any areas in which you feel you need more work, let your counselor know. Remember, it's best to be completely prepared to manage the high-risk situations that can lead to relapse and/or ineffective chronic pain management.

Good luck on your journey of effective pain management and recovery!

Take a few minutes to complete this exercise in your APM workbook.

Although the above exercise can be an effective benchmark for you to evaluate yourself, follow-up sessions with a counselor or therapist are needed for tune-ups and to determine the ongoing effectiveness of your treatment. Some of you may also benefit from completing a Relapse Prevention Therapy process.

A New Beginning

Using the APM modality increases positive treatment outcomes.

The Road Map to APM Recovery

As you have seen, APM recovery uses detailed, accurate assessments followed by multidimensional treatment plans. These treatment plans include the *core clinical processes*, and when needed the *medication management components* and the *holistic treatment processes*. Proven CENAPS® relapse prevention methods are implemented to help ensure ongoing recovery.

An Integrated APM Treatment Approach
- Core Clinical Processes
- Medication Management Components
- Holistic Treatment Processes

Using the APM system leads to a more positive outcome than from either traditional chemical dependency treatment or pain-management care at a chronic pain clinic, thus enabling you to resume a healthy and productive life.

This was the case for Donna. She was able to stop all of her problematic pain medication. Her relationships with her husband and family also improved. In addition, she continued to build trust and safety in her women's group and is working an effective pain management program.

Donna didn't relapse, but her life did become very stressful and she needed to backtrack into some basic self-care treatment planning. In addition, she was encouraged to start working on relapse prevention therapy as soon as possible.

Matt, unfortunately, continues to struggle. He is much more hopeful, however, that he will eventually succeed in becoming a high-functioning member of society again. His prognosis has significantly improved as a result of the APM process. He should become totally stabilized and move into healthy, ongoing recovery, based on his current signs of progress. He also needs to complete a relapse prevention therapy process in order to manage his core psychological issues.

Spreading the Word—APM Works

Congratulations for finishing this book and the APM workbook. You are now a part of the APM system. This is a new beginning. It's up to you to help continue the work to further develop your personalized APM recovery and relapse prevention plan. You can do this by practicing what you have learned and sharing your progress with other people in chronic pain.

Appendix

Introducing Dr. Mark Stanford

Because of his unique qualifications, I asked Mark Stanford, Ph.D., to contribute his expertise in explaining the physiology of pain sensation and the pharmacological implications for determining the proper medication for ongoing chronic pain conditions. The foundation for the chapter one section on pain in the *Addiction-Free Pain Management Professional Guide* was developed by referring to Dr. Stanford's book, *Foundations in Behavioral Pharmacology*, as well as Addiction-Free Pain Management classes we taught together, and the paper he wrote on the "Neurophysiology of Pain."

Dr. Stanford has a clinical background in substance-abuse health care and community mental health spanning almost twenty years. He has published numerous materials on the biochemical basis of behavior and addictive disorders and has addressed audiences throughout the nation. He is president and CEO of PharmTech, a research and consultant group in behavioral health.

He is an educator in the neurosciences and a professor of psychopharmacology at San Jose State University. Dr. Stanford also lectures on addiction medicine and pharmacology at Stanford University School of Medicine, U.C. Berkeley Extension, and JFK University in San Jose, California.

Medical Marijuana Controversy

By Stephen F. Grinstead, M.A., ACRPS

Although we have entered a new millennium many old controversies are still raging. One of these issues is the use of marijuana as a legitimate medication. There are two polarized camps fueling this debate. One side preaches the evils of using this herb and the other side extols the virtues.

Over the past two decades I have listened to both sides of this issue and have seen the impact of this controversy on my clients. Unfortunately, there is an important piece missing; reliable double-blind studies designed to test how effective marijuana really is as a legitimate medication. There is also the issue of how the U.S. Drug Enforcement Agency (DEA) rates or "schedules" drugs.

What has been available for several years as a legitimate medication is Marinol[R] (dronabinol), a synthetic THC (the active psychoactive chemical in marijuana). While marijuana is still listed as a Schedule I drug by the DEA and illegal for medical use, Marinol (the synthetic form of THC) has finally been reduced from a Schedule II to a Schedule III drug.

For Schedule I substances, the criteria that need to be considered are whether the substance has a high potential for abuse, has no currently accepted medical use in treatment in the United States, and has a lack of accepted safety for use under medical supervision. While Schedule I drugs cannot be used medically, the law does allow supervised research.

For substances in Schedule II, the criteria that need to be considered are its high potential for abuse, whether it has a currently accepted medical use in treatment in the United States or a currently accepted medical use with severe restrictions and whether abuse of the substances may lead to severe psychological or physical dependence. While legal for medical use, doctors need to go through additional legal steps when prescribing these drugs.

A substance is placed on Schedule III based on its potential for abuse relative to substances in other schedules, whether it has a currently accepted medical use in treatment in the United States, and its relative potential to produce physical or psychological dependence is less.

Marinol has been used in treating glaucoma, people undergoing chemotherapy, and for AIDS patients. Again sides are split on the effectiveness of this medication. One side says Marinol works great, therefore there is no need to legalize the medical use of marijuana. The other side states that Marinol is not nearly as effective as smoked marijuana.

After working with many individuals who have used Marinol and also smoked marijuana, I see that both sides have some good points. For example, after helping some of my clients work through denial issues surrounding marijuana abuse, they become honest and share that the Marinol did work as well for controlling nausea or increasing appetite, but they didn't get high. On the other hand, several clients who needed help for nausea caused by chemotherapy treatment were not able to ingest the Marinol tablets and found smoking marijuana to be a much better option.

The major problems I have with smoking marijuana as a medicine is the inability to regulate the dosage and, even more important, the delivery system. The level of THC varies so greatly in the marijuana that is currently available that coming up with a therapeutic dose is extremely difficult. In addition, the marijuana has other ingredients that may have unfortunate side effects. Then there is the dangerous delivery system—the issue of smoking it. No other medication we have is administered that way because of the potential dangers.

Because of the lack of research there has been no exploration of a safer delivery system for the active ingredient of marijuana (THC). There have been suggestions that an aerosol delivery system for the THC or Marinol would eliminate the dosage and the unsafe smoking problems. Why is this not being given due consideration?

One of the reasons may be that there is not enough profit for drug companies, but I believe the main reason is the stigma that has historically surrounded marijuana. I do believe that marijuana is a serious drug of abuse that leads to dependency (addiction) but this is also true of many legal prescription medications. For example Vicodin[R] and OxyContin[R] have both been increasingly abused in the past several years, and Valium[R] (diazepam) and Xanax[R] (alprazolam) have been a serious abuse problem for at least the past decade.

Another problem with medical marijuana is that oftentimes it is being prescribed for conditions that may not be medially indicated. In fact, several of my clients received prescriptions for stress management and pain management.

I am not aware of any legitimate research that indicates marijuana is a medically sound treatment for either of those conditions. That is why quality research needs to be undertaken to prove once and for all the legitimacy of using marijuana—or at least its active ingredient THC—to treat specific medical conditions.

I do understand this is a controversial issue. While I am not in favor of legalizing "street drugs," I do advocate utilizing a potentially effective medication after it has undergone the same level of testing as the other medications we currently use. However, I believe that in addition to verifying the effectiveness, the delivery system and dosage problems also need to be resolved before I would feel comfortable endorsing the use of medicinal marijuana.

Pain References

Catalano, E. and K. Hardin. *The Chronic Pain Control Workbook: A Step-by-Step Guide for Coping with and Overcoming Pain*. Oakland, California: New Harbinger, 1996.

Caudill, M. *Managing Pain Before It Manages You*. New York: Guilford Press, 1995, revised 2001.

Cleveland, M. *Living Well: A Twelve-Step Response to Chronic Illness and Disability*. Center City, Minnesota: Hazelden, 1988.

Corey, A., G. Linssen, and P. Spinhoven. "Multimodal Treatment Programs for Chronic Pain: A Quantitative Analysis of Existing Research Data," *Journal of Psychosomatic Research* 36, no. 3 (1992): 275–286.

Corey, D. and S. Solomon. *Pain: Free Yourself for Life*. New York: Penguin Books, 1989.

Davis, M., E. R. Eshelman, and M. McKay. *The Relaxation & Stress Reduction Workbook (4th Edition)*. Oakland, California: New Harbinger, 1995.

Deardorff, W., A. Chino, and D. Scott. "Characteristics of Chronic Pain Patients: Factor Analysis of the MMPI-2," *Pain* 54, no. 1 (1993): 153–158.

Deardorff, W., H. Rubin, and D. Scott. "Comprehensive Multidisciplinary Treatment of Chronic Pain: A Follow-up Study of Treated and Non-treated Groups," *Pain* 45, no. 1 (1991): 35–43.

Egoscue, P. *Pain Free: A Revolutionary Method for Stopping Chronic Pain*. New York: Bantam, 1998.

Ford, N. *Painstoppers: The Magic of All-Natural Pain Relief*. West Nyack, New York: Parker, 1994.

Fuhr, A. "Activator Methods Chiropractic Technique: The Science and Art," *Today's Chiropractic* (July/August 1995): 48–52.

Grinstead, S. and T. Gorski. *Addiction-Free Pain Management: The Professional Guide.* Independence, Missouri: Herald House/Independence Press, 1999.

Grinstead, S. and T. Gorski. *Addiction-Free Pain Management: Relapse Prevention Counseling Workbook.* Independence, Missouri: Herald House/Independence Press, 1997.

Halpern, L. and J. Robinson. "Prescribing Practices for Pain in Drug Dependence: A Lesson in Ignorance," *Advances in Alcohol and Substance Abuse* 5, no. 1–2 (1986): 135–162.

Jaffe, D. *Healing from Within: Psychological Techniques You Can Use to Help the Mind Heal the Body.* New York: Simon and Schuster, 1986.

Kennedy, J. and T. Crowley. "Chronic Pain and Substance Abuse: A Pilot Study of Opioid Maintenance," *Journal of Substance Abuse Treatment* 7, no. 4 (1990): 233–238.

Kingdon, R., K. Stanley, and R. Kizior. *Handbook for Pain Management.* Philadelphia, Pennsylvania: W. B. Saunders, 1998.

Linchitz, R. *Life Without Pain: Free Yourself from Chronic Back Pain, Headache, Arthritis Pain, and More, Without Surgery or Narcotic Drugs.* New York: Addison-Wesly Publishing, 1987.

Meade, T., et al. "Randomized Comparison of Chiropractic and Hospital Outpatient Management for Low Back Pain: Results from Extended Follow-up," *British Medical Journal* 311 (1995): 349–351.

Milne, E. "The Mechanism and Treatment of Migraine and Other Disorders of Cervical and Postural Dysfunction," *Cephalaalgia* 9 supplement, No. 10 (1989): 381–382.

Murray, M. *The Healing Power of Herbs: The Enlightened Person's Guide to the Wonders of Medicinal Plants,* 2nd Edition. Rocklin, California: Prima Publishing, 1995.

Murray, M. and J. Pizzorno. *Encyclopedia of Natural Medicine*. Rocklin, California: Prima Publishing, 1991.

Osterbauer, P., et al. "Three-Dimensional Head Kinetics and Clinical Outcome of Patients with Neck Injury Treated with Manipulative Therapy: A Pilot Study," *Journal of Manipulative Physiological Therapy* 15, no. 8 (1992): 501–511.

Reilly, R. *Living With Pain: A New Approach to the Management of Chronic Pain*. Minneapolis, Minnesota: Deaconess, 1993.

Rogers, R. and C. McMillin. *The Healing Bond: Treating Addictions in Groups*. New York: W.W. Norton & Company, 1989.

Roy, R. *The Social Contex of the Chronic Pain Sufferer*. Toronto, Canada: University of Toronto Press, 1992.

Sarno, J. *Healing Back Pain: The Mind Body Connection*. New York: Warner Books, 1991.

Sarno, J. *The Mind Body Prescription: Healing the Body, Healing the Pain*. New York: Warner Books, 1998.

Stacy, C., A. Kaplan, and G. Williams. *The Fight Against Pain*. New York: Consumers Union, 1992.

Stanford, M. *Foundations in Behavioral Pharmacology: For Social Workers, Psychologists, Therapists, and Counselors*. Santa Cruz, California: Lightway Centre, 1998.

Stimmel, B. *Pain, Analgesics, and Addictions*. New York: Raven, 1983.

Stimmel, B. *Pain and Its Relief without Addiction*. New York: Haworth Medical, 1997.

Tennant, F., J. Shannon, J. Nork, A. Sagherian, and M. Berman. "Abnormal Adrenal Gland Metabolism in Opioid Addicts: Implications for Clinical Treatment," *Journal of Psychoactive Drugs* 23, no. 2 (1991): 135–149.

Turk, D., T. Rudy, and B. Sorkin. "Neglected Topics in Chronic Pain Treatment Outcome Studies: Determination of Success," *Pain* 53, no. 1 (1993): 3–16.

Vertosick, F. *Why We Hurt: The Natural History of Pain.* New York: Harcourt, 2000.

Wall, P. and M. Jones. *Defeating Pain: The War Against the Silent Epidemic.* New York: Plenum, 1991.

Warfield, C. *Expert Pain Management.* Spring House, Pennsylvania: Springhouse, 1996.

Relapse Prevention References

Gorski, Terence T, and Merlene Miller. *Counseling for Relapse Prevention*. Independence, Missouri: Herald House/Independence Press, 1982.

Gorski, Terence T. and Merlene Miller. *Staying Sober: A Guide for Relapse Prevention*. Independence, Missouri: Herald House/Independence Press, 1986.

Gorski, Terence T. *The Staying Sober Workbook: A Serious Solution for the Problem of Relapse*. Independence, Missouri: Herald House/Independence Press, 1988.

Gorski, Terence T. *Do Family of Origin Problems Cause Chemical Addiction?* Independence, Missouri: Herald House/Independence Press, 1989.

Gorski, Terence T. *How to Start Relapse Prevention Support Groups*. Independence, Missouri: Herald House/Independence Press, 1989.

Gorski, Terence T. *Passages Through Recovery: An Action Plan for Preventing Relapse*. Center City, Minnesota: Hazelden, 1989.

Gorski, Terence T. *The Players and Their Personalities.* Independence, Missouri: Herald House/Independence Press, 1989.

Gorski, Terence T. *Understanding the Twelve Steps: A Guide for Counselors, Therapists, and Recovering People.* Independence, Missouri: Herald House/Independence Press, 1989.

Gorski, Terence T. *Understanding the Twelve Steps: An Interpretation and Guide for Recovering People.* New York: Prentice Hall Press, 1989.

Gorski, Terence T. *Keeping the Balance: A Psychospiritual Model of Growth and Development.* Independence, Missouri: Herald House/Independence Press, 1993.

Gorski, Terence T. *Part Two: Relapse Prevention Therapy with Chemically Dependent Criminal Offenders—A Guide for Counselors, Therapists, and Criminal Justice Professionals.* Independence, Missouri: Herald House/Independence Press, 1994.

Gorski, Terence T. *A Group Leader's Guide to Brief, Strategic Problem-Solving Group Therapy.* Independence, Missouri: Herald House/Independence Press, 1995.

Gorski, Terence T. *A Group Member's Guide to Brief, Strategic Problem-Solving Group Therapy.* Independence, Missouri: Herald House/Independence Press, 1995.

Gorski, Terence T. with Stephen F. Grinstead. *Denial Management Counseling Workbook.* Independence, Missouri: Herald House/Independence Press, 2000.

Gorski, Terence T. with Stephen F. Grinstead. *Denial Management Counseling Professional Guide.* Independence, Missouri: Herald House/Independence Press, 1995.

Grinstead, Stephen F. and Terence T. Gorski. *Food Addiction: Recovery and Relapse Prevention Workbook for Compulsive Overeaters, Binge Eaters, and Food Addicts.* Independence, Missouri: Herald House/Independence Press, 2001.

Marlatt, G. Alan. *Relapse Prevention: Maintenance Strategies in the Treatment of Addictive Behaviors.* New York: Guilford Press, 1985.

Miller, Merlene, Terence T. Gorski, and David Miller. *Learning to Live Again: A Guide for Recovery from Alcoholism.* Independence, Missouri: Herald House/Independence Press, 1980.

Miller, Merlene and Terence T. Gorski. *Family Recovery: Growing Beyond Addiction.* Independence, Missouri: Herald House/Independence Press, 1982.

Miller, Merlene and Terence T. Gorski. *Staying Sober Recovery Education Modules—Exercise Manual.* Independence, Missouri: Herald House/Independence Press, 1989.

Miller, Merlene and Terence T. Gorski. *Staying Sober Recovery Education Modules.* Independence, Missouri: Herald House/Independence Press, 1989.

Booklets and Pamphlets

Gorski, Terence T. and Merlene Miller. *The Relapse Dynamic.* Independence, Missouri: Herald House/Independence Press, 1980.

Gorski, Terence T. and Merlene Miller. *The Phases and Warning Signs of Relapse.* Independence, Missouri: Herald House/Independence Press, 1984.

Gorski, Terence T. and Merlene Miller. *Mistaken Beliefs About Relapse.* Independence, Missouri: Herald House/Independence Press, 1988.

Gorski, Terence T. *The Relapse Recovery Grid.* Center City, Minnesota: Hazelden, 1989.

Gorski, Terence T. and Merlene Miller. *Understanding Addictive Disease.* Independence, Missouri: Herald House/Independence Press, 1990.

Gorski, Terence T. *Questionnaire of Twelve Step Completion.* Independence, Missouri: Herald House/Independence Press, 1990.

Gorski, Terence T. *Relapse Warning Signs for Criminal Behavior.* Independence, Missouri: Herald House/Independence Press, 1994.

Gorski, Terence T. *The Relapse Dynamic for Criminal Behavior.* Independence, Missouri: Herald House/Independence Press, 1994.

Gorski, Terence T. *Biopsychosocial Model of Alcoholism and Drug Addiction: Lecture Notes.* Independence, Missouri: Herald House/Independence Press, 1999.

Miller, Merlene and Terence T. Gorski. *Lowering the Risk: A Self-Care Plan for Relapse Prevention.* Independence, Missouri: Herald House/Independence Press, 1990.